Therapeutic Radiology for the House Officer

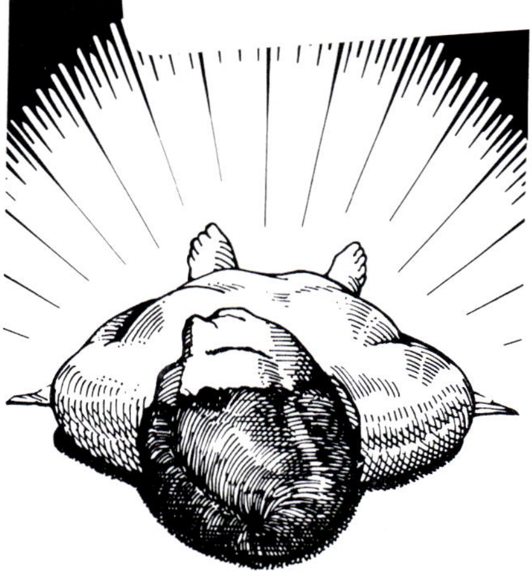

Therapeutic Radiology for the House Officer

Lawrence R. Coia, M.D.
Assistant Professor
Department of Radiation Therapy
University of Pennsylvania School of Medicine
Fox Chase Cancer Center
Philadelphia, Pennsylvania

David J. Moylan, III, M.D.
Assistant Professor
Department of Radiation Therapy and Nuclear Medicine
Thomas Jefferson University
Philadelphia, Pennsylvania

with a foreword by
Simon Kramer, M.D.
Distinguished Professor
Department of Radiation Therapy and Nuclear Medicine
Thomas Jefferson University
Philadelphia, Pennsylvania

WILLIAMS & WILKINS
Baltimore/London

Editor: George Stamathis
Associate Editor: Jonathan W. Pine, Jr.
Design: JoAnne Janowiak
Illustration Planning: Joseph P. Cummings
Production: Carol Eckhart

Library of Congress Cataloging in Publication Data

Coia, Lawrence R.
Therapeutic radiology for the house officer.

Includes index.
1. Cancer—Radiotherapy. I. Moylan, David J. II. Title.
RC271.R3C64 1984 616.99′40642 84-2397
INBS 0-683-02051-X

Composed and printed at the Waverly Press, Inc.
Mt. Royal and Guilford Aves.
Baltimore, MD 21202, U.S.A.

Dedication

To our parents for all their encouragement and support.

Foreword

One of the best kept secrets in medicine is the fact that of all the chronic diseases, cancer is today the most curable. Of the 730,000 patients with invasive cancer seen each year, 40% are cured by surgery, radiation therapy and chemotherapy or by appropriate combinations of these modalities. Apart from the acute surgical episode, most potentially curable cancer patients are treated on an ambulatory basis, and since in most medical schools students and residents have little contact with outpatients, it is not surprising that this group of patients escapes their attention. On the other hand, patients with recurrent and advanced malignant disease are frequently admitted to the hospital and, thus, both students and residents are exposed primarily to the incurable cancer patient and hence in their formative years develop the attitude that cancer management is a depressing and unrewarding field.

One-half of all cancer patients in the United States receive radiation therapy at one time or another during the course of their disease, and one-half of these patients are potentially curable. Yet, the non-specialist is rarely exposed to the discipline of radiation therapy and even those who develop an interest in oncology have little understanding of our field.

Doctors Coia and Moylan have undertaken to develop a handbook which will explain the concepts and rationale of radiation therapy in the various areas where radiation therapy has a major impact on the cancer patient. They de-emphasized techniques of irradiation and have instead dealt with those aspects that can lead to an understanding of where and how radiation therapy can be useful. They describe the clinical and laboratory investigations needed to arrive at a treatment decision and discuss the pros and cons of radiation therapy, site by site. In order to let the reader decide the usefulness of this treatment in a specific case, data on outcome and complications are presented in a similar way.

Most physicians, in whatever branch of medicine, will be called upon to advise and make decisions on patients with malignant disease. I hope that this volume will give residents, house officers and medical students a better understanding of our field and allow them to participate intelligently in the inital treatment decision. This initial decision so often determines success or failure in the management of cancer patients.

Simon Kramer, M.D.

About the Authors

Lawrence R. Coia, M.D., M.A., is currently Assistant Professor of Radiation Therapy at the University of Pennsylvania School of Medicine and Attending Radiotherapist at the Fox Chase Cancer Center. He was formerly Chief Resident in Radiation Therapy at Thomas Jefferson University Hospital. He attended Rensselaer Polytechnic Institute, the Swiss Federal Institute of Technology, the Bryn Mawr Graduate School of Sciences and Temple University School of Medicine. His research interests include neutron beam therapy and combined-modality treatment for esophageal carcinoma.

David J. Moylan, III, M.D., is Assistant Professor of Radiation Therapy and Nuclear Medicine at Jefferson Medical College of Thomas Jefferson University, where he was also a former Chief Resident in Radiation Therapy. Dr. Moylan graduated from the Massachussetts Institute of Technology and Georgetown University School of Medicine. He completed two years of residency training in Internal Medicine at the Bryn Mawr Hospital. He is presently an Attending Physician at Thomas Jefferson University Hospital and consultant at Wills Eye Hospital. He is a recipient of the American Cancer Society Junior Faculty Clinical Fellowship. His research activities include hyperthermia and radioimmunoglobulin therapy.

With a foreword by Simon Kramer, M.D.

Simon Kramer, M.D., is Distinguished Professor of Radiation Therapy and Nuclear Medicine at Jefferson Medical College of Thomas Jefferson University. He has served as head of Radiation Therapy at Thomas Jefferson University Hospital from 1956 through 1983. Dr. Kramer is a graduate of King's College and King's College Hospital Medical School, University of London, London, England. He served in the British Medical Corps from 1943-1947. He completed training in radiation therapy at Meyerstein Institute of Radiotherapy Middlesex Hospital, University of London, London, England. In

1971, Dr. Kramer helped found the Radiation Therapy Oncology Group, RTOG, a nationwide cooperative group investigating the role of radiotherapy in various malignancies. He is also principal investigator of the Patterns of Care Study, designed to establish benchmarks of the quality of radiation therapy in the United States. Dr. Kramer has authored over 150 articles dealing with the science of radiation therapy and is a world-renowned authority in neuro-oncology and the therapy of head and neck tumors.

Preface

A substantial proportion of admissions to a general hospital are to investigate patients with signs or symptoms that may be cancer-related. Examples of this abound: anemia, a solitary pulmonary nodule, hematuria, hematochezia or post-menopausal bleeding. Once a diagnosis of cancer has been established, approximately 50% of patients will receive radiation therapy at some time during their course either as curative, adjuvant or palliative treatment. Therefore, it is important for house officers in the various subspecialties of internal medicine and surgery, who are responsible for the care of these patients, to have a rudimentary knowledge of radiation therapy in order to evaluate what therapeutic response and morbidity can be expected from its application.

This manual is organized to be clinically useful. In the introductory chapters on radiation physics and radiobiology, important terms and concepts used in clinical radiotherapy are covered. The subsequent chapters, which form the core of the handbook, group tumors predominantly according to major physiologic systems or anatomic site. Admittedly, this approach is somewhat arbitrary and artificial but hopefully expedient. Usually, for each tumor a brief overview is presented followed by a review of pathology, staging, work-up, clinical features, management, results of therapy and morbidity. In the morbidity sections, acute and chronic complications of treatment are listed along with pertinant information regarding their pathogenesis and management. There are also chapters dealing with radiotherapeutic emergencies, palliative treatment and combined-modality therapy. The Radiation Safety chapter presents guidelines for radiation protection. Current areas of promising investigation are presented in the final chapter.

The index is comprehensive and is intended to be useful in quickly locating important terms. This extensive index avoids the necessity of repeating new terms and definitions in a glossary or appendix. In keeping with the theme of the house officer series, the thrust of this manual is a practical and common sense approach to the patient receiving radiation therpay. Hopefully, it will enable house officers to interact more effectively with the therapeutic radiologist. We feel this handbook may have more general appeal to anyone involved in cancer patient care and may be particularly useful to medical students, residents, and fellows in medical oncology, gynecologic oncology and head and neck surgery and may serve as an introduction to first year residents in radiation oncology.

Lawrence R. Coia, M.D.

Lawrence R. Coia, M.D.

David J. Moylan III, M.D.

David J. Moylan III, M.D.

Acknowledgements

The authors wish to express their special thanks to Terri Anderson without whose patient secretarial assistance this manual would not be possible. We would also like to thank Sophia Grzbowski, Debbie Summers and Gina Strecker, who also assisted in manuscript preparation. We gratefully acknowledge the help and encouragement of our colleagues who reviewed parts of the manuscript:

Darryl Brown, Ph.D., Barbara Danoff, M.D., Jerome Derdel, M.D., Ben Galkin, M.S., Michael Gallagher, M.D., Robert Goodman, M.D., Mahroo Haghbin, M.D., Simon Kramer, M.D., Mohammed Mohiuddin, M.D., Melvyn Richter, M.D., Nagalingam Suntharalingam, Ph.D., and Richard Yelovich, M.D. We are also grateful to Barbara Schreiber-Coia for providing the comprehensive index.

The assistance of editorial staff members of the Williams & Wilkins Company including Alice Reid, Jonathan Pine and George Stamathis was instrumental in bringing this project to fruition.

Contents

Chapter 1

Physics of Therapeutic Radiology

OVERVIEW

Since radiotherapists make use of ionizing radiation to eradicate malignancies, it is important to understand what this type of radiation is, how it is produced, how it interacts in tissue and how it can be effectively administered in treating malignancies. Ionizing radiation is comprised of electromagnetic and particulate radiation (See Figure 1.1). Apart from the use of electrons, most of radiation therapy is based on the use of electromagnetic radiation (also called photons).

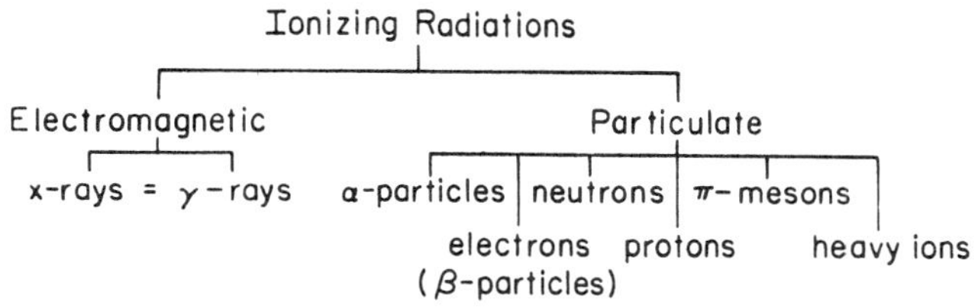

Figure 1.1. Ionizing radiation.

IONIZING ELECTROMAGNETIC RADIATION

The electromagnetic energy spectrum ranges from low energy radiowaves of long wavelength and low frequency to high energy ionizing radiation of short wavelength and high frequency (See Figure 1.2). The high energy end of the spectrum comprises ionizing radiation. From the direct relationship between energy (E) and frequency (γ)

$$E = h\gamma$$

h = Planck's constant (6.625 x 10^{-27} erg-sec)

and the inverse relationship of frequency (γ) and wavelength (γ)

$$c = \gamma\lambda$$

c = speed of light (3 x 10^8 m/sec)

one can derive a simple relation between energy (expressed in KeV*) and wavelength (expressed in Angstroms):

$$E = 12.4/\lambda$$

For example, radiation with a wavelength of one A corresponds to radiation energy of 12.4 KeV. Although ionization can occur with energies of under 100 eV, most of radiation therapy is based on radiation of energies between 10 KeV and 100 MeV.

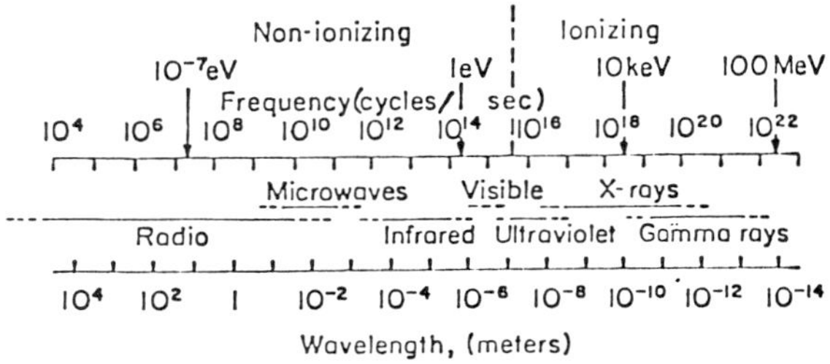

Figure 1.2. The electromagnectic spectrum. Energy increases from left to right. Selected energies are shown.

* An electron volt (eV) is a unit of energy representing the amount of energy acquired by an electron accelerated through 1 volt. A KeV equals 1000 electron volts.

When high energy radiation interacts with matter, electrons are removed from their atomic or molecular orbits, resulting in ionization. On the average about 33 eV per ionization in air is released, which is a significant amount of energy at the atomic and molecular level.

X-rays and gamma rays are both types of ionizing radiation. They are intrinsically the same except for the way that they are produced.

X-rays

X-rays are obtained from extra-nuclear processes. For instance, when an accelerated electron strikes a target, it is slowed down by the nuclei of the target material and during the deceleration x-rays (or bremstrahlung) are emitted. This is the process used to produce most useful radiation from x-ray units, accelerators and betatrons.

X-rays can also be produced when an orbital electron is removed from an atom. X-rays are then emitted when subsequent electrons in other orbitals lose energy as they cascade into the vacancies created. Such radiation is called characteristic radiation since the radiation emitted is characteristic of the element whose electrons have been removed.

Gamma-rays

Gamma radiation is obtained from intranuclear processes. Radioactive isotopic decay occurs when an unstable nucleus gives off excess energy in the form of gamma radiation in decaying to a more stable form. Radioactive isotopic decay occurs exponentially as a function of time. The half-life of a radioisotope represents the time needed for it to decay from a given activity to one-half of that activity. The activity of a radioisotope is the number of decays it undergoes per second and is measured in curies, or, more recently, in bequerels. An activity of one curie (Ci) is equal to 3.7 x 1010 disintegrations per second. A bequerel (Bq) is equal to one disintegration per second.

IONIZING PARTICULATE RADIATION

Atomic constituents can also be used to produce ionization. These include electrons, protons, alpha particles, neutrons, negative pi mesons and heavy ions. At present, only electrons are commonly used in radiotherapy. The radiotherapeutic value of other particulate radiations is under investigation. Electrons, because of their charge and low mass, can be accelerated to high energies by means of an electrical device such as a linear accelerator or a betatron. Electrons are also produced during nuclear decay (beta decay) and are referred to as beta-particles. Unlike X and gamma radiation which are absorbed exponentially in matter, electrons have a finite range.

INTERACTION OF RADIATION IN TISSUE

Radiation is scattered and absorbed in tissue. The intensity of a beam incident on tissue is attenuated exponentially.

$$I = I_o e^{-\mu t}$$

Where:

- I_o - incident intensity
- I - emergent intensity
- μ - absorption coefficient (for a mono energetic beam in a specific tissue)
- t - thickness of tissue

The relative amount of radiation emerging is dependent on the absorption coefficient of the tissue (μ) and its thickness (t). Three major types of interaction occur between radiation and matter which determine the absorption coefficient:

1. The Photoelectric Effect - Radiation is absorbed by an innermost orbital electron resulting in the electron's ejection from the atom. This effect predominates at low energies (less than 35 KeV) and is highly dependent on the atomic number (Z) of the absorbing material. This effect accounts for the use of lead and other high Z materials in absorbing low energy ionizing radiation. Also, it results in bone absorbing more radiation than soft tissue, the basis for diagnostic radiology.

2. The Compton Effect - Incoming radiation is scattered by loosely bound electrons which themselves are ejected from the atom. This process is the most important means of absorption of ionizing radiation in radiation therapy. It predominates in tissue over a wide energy range (35 KeV - 50 MeV). It is independent of the atomic number of the absorbing material and thus a given amount of incident radiation is roughly absorbed to the same extent gram for gram whether the material be soft tissue or bone.

3. Pair Production - Radiation energy is transformed into a pair of particles -- an electron and a positron (a positively charged electron). Pair production has a threshold energy of 1.02 MeV, becomes important in the high energy range (>10 MeV), and is dependent on atomic number.

Inverse Square Law: The intensity (I) of a beam of radiation is inversely proportional to the square of the distance (d) from a point source:

$$I \propto 1/d^2$$

This relation is very important in radiation protection (See Chapter 19) as well as in radiotherapy.

When short treatment distances are utilized in radiotherapy, a rapid fall off in dose with distance is noted due to the inverse square relation. Such a situation occurs with brachytherapy and also with superficial external beam radiotherapy. Brachy means short distance thus brachytherapy means therapy with a short distance between the radiation source and the target (as with radioisotope implants). Most high energy external beam radiation therapy is given at long (teletherapy) treatment distances of 80-120 cm, so that the fall off in dose with distance is relatively small.

RADIATION MEASUREMENTS

The quantity of radiation measurement of fundamental use in radiation therapy is the amount of energy absorbed from a beam of radiation per unit mass of absorbing material. This quantity is referred to as the absorbed dose. The rad is the most commonly used unit and represents 100 ergs absorbed per gram. Another unit currently recommended for usage is the gray (Gy), which represents one joule absorbed per kg. (Note: 1 gray = 100 rad and 1 centigray = 1 rad). When one rad is given to tissue, the same amount of energy per unit mass is given irrespective of the type of radiation or the type of absorbing tissue. For each rad given, each gram of tissue will absorb an energy of 100 erg.

Unfortunately, direct measurement of absorbed dose is difficult and impractical. Instead, the amount of ionization produced by a beam of radiation in air is measured and is referred to as radiation exposure. The unit of exposure is the roentgen (R)*. From this quantity and knowledge of the energy of the radiation and absorption coefficient of the absorbing tissue, we can compute the absorbed dose. For example, in the high energy range which is commonly used in radiation therapy (>1 MeV), one roentgen of exposure in air represents approximately 0.95 rad absorbed dose in tissue.

*One roentgen = 2.58×10^{-4} coulomb/kg air

RADIATION SOURCES

External beam units deliver radiation from a unit external to the patient, such as an x-ray machine, a linear accelerator, a betatron or a radioisotopic Cobalt 60 unit (See Figure 1.3). Radiation emitted from x-ray units and radioisotope sources may be characterized by their penetrating power. The thickness of absorber needed to reduce the beam intensity by one-half is referred to as the half value layer (HVL) and is expressed in millimeters (or centimeters) of the absorber, usually copper, lead or aluminum. High energy beams are often characterized by their maximum energy and by the depth in tissue at which 50% of the dose is delivered (See Table 1.2).

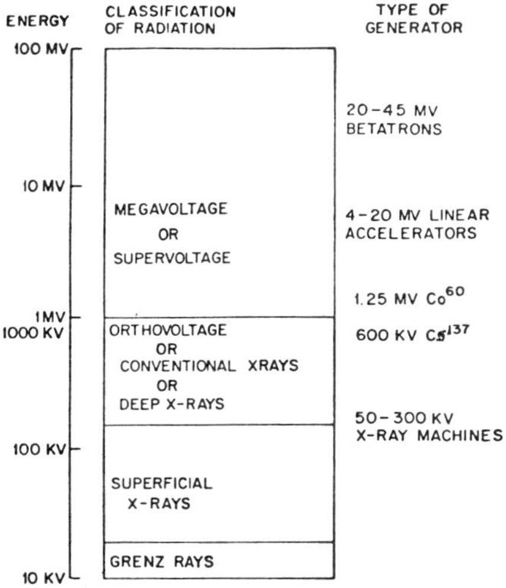

Figure 1.3. External beam units.

Brachytherapy sources are usually radioisotopes which are placed into the tumor (interstitial therapy) or near the tumor in a body cavity (intracavitary therapy). Important characteristics of radioisotopes used in brachytherapy include their half-life, energies emitted and half-value layer.

Table 1.1 lists characteristics of frequently used radioisotopes in brachytherapy. (Cobalt 60 is rarely used in brachytherapy but is an important teletherapy source).

Table 1.1
Characteristics of Frequently Used Radioisotopes

Radio-Isotope	Half-life	γ-Radiation avg. E (MEV)	HVL in Lead (cm)
Cobalt 60	5.3 yrs.	1.25	1.2
Cesium 137	30 yrs.	0.661	0.6
Iridium 192	74 days	0.350	0.6
Gold 198	2.7 days	0.412	0.3
Radon 222	3.8 days	0.047-2.4	1.66
Radium 226	1622 yrs.	0.047-2.4	1.66
Iodine 125	60 days	0.028	0.003

EXTERNAL BEAM UNITS (See Figure 1.3)

X-ray machines: Electrons emitted from a hot filament are accelerated onto a tungsten target and produce x-rays. Beams from these units are not monoenergetic. A spectrum of x-rays are produced with a maximum energy equal to the maximum energy of the accelerated electrons and an average energy of about one third of the maximum. Grenz rays are very low energy x-rays from 10 to 30 KeV. Superficial units produce x-ray energies of 30 to 125 KeV, while the maximum energy range of orthovoltage units is between 125 and 500 KeV.

Linear accelerators and betatrons: Energies above 1 MeV, referred to as supervoltage or megavoltage energies, are easily attained with these units. A linear accelerator accelerates electrons along a linear path in a wave guide. In a betatron, a changing magnetic field accelerates the electrons along a circular orbit. In either unit, these electrons may be extracted directly for electron treatment or they may be directed onto a target to produce high energy x-rays. Like x-ray machines, a spectrum of x-ray energies is produced with a maximum energy limited by the accelerating potential. Unlike superficial and some orthovoltage radiation, the absorption of megavoltage radiation is relatively independent of the absorbing tissue, since the Compton effect, rather than the photoelectric effect, predominates. This fact, coupled with a greater degree of penetration and skin sparing, makes megavoltage radiation treatment a very important tool for radiotherapists. (See Table 1.2)

Table 1.2
Skin Sparing and Depth at 50% Dose for Commonly Used External XRT Beams

Maximum Beam Energy	Depth of Dose Maximum	50% Depth Dose (10 X 10 cm field)
250 KeV (x-ray unit)	Surface	7 cm
1.25 MeV (^{60}Co)	0.5 cm	11 cm
Linear Accelerators		
4 MeV	1.0 cm	14 cm
6 MeV	1.5 cm	16 cm
10 MeV	2.0 cm	18 cm
15 MeV	3.0 cm	20 cm
Betatrons		
25 MeV	4.0 cm	23 cm
35 MeV	5.0 cm	26 cm

Cobalt 60: Cobalt 60 is an artificial radioactive isotope that produces radiation useful in radiotherapy. When Co 60 decays to Ni 60, it produces gamma radiation of 1.117 and 1.33 MeV (average of 1.25 MeV). By housing this radioactive source in a bulky lead treatment head, the isotropically emitted radiation can be collimated into a treatment beam. Cobalt units have advantages over orthovoltage units, including skin sparing and

better beam penetration. Since cobalt units are less complex than betatrons or accelerators, they often require less maintenance. The half-life of Co 60 is approximately five years and thus sources must be replaced every several years to avoid very low beam outputs. A disadvantage of a cobalt unit compared to accelerators and betatrons is that because a relatively large radioisotope source must be used, the edge of the treatment field is not as sharply defined due to the larger penumbra associated with the cobalt source size. Also, the depth of penetration may not be as good. (See Figure 1.4).

Depth Dose Curves

The depth dose curve reflects the percentage of the maximum dose delivered as a function of depth within the absorbing material (usually water or tissue). The relative depth dose distribution for several types of radiation beams are shown in Figure 1.4. Note the increase in tissue penetration and skin sparing with higher energies (also illustrated in Table 1.2). Depth dose distributions are also dependent on a number of other factors besides beam energy such as the field size and the distance between the radiation source and absorbing material.

The electron dose profile in Figure 1.4 shows a limited range of penetration. <u>Note that the range of an electron in centimeters is approximately one-half the energy in MeV.</u> Also, the depth, in centimeters, at which 80% of the maximum dose is given is approximately 1/3 of the electron energy in MeV. For example, a 12 MeV electron has a range of 6 cm and 80% of the maximum dose is at 4 cm.

By combining electron and photon beams in a one to one ratio, a <u>mixed beam</u> will result which has depth dose characteristics intermediate between these two beams. This technique is useful in treatment planning to deliver an optimal dose at intermediaite depths with sparing of deep tissues.

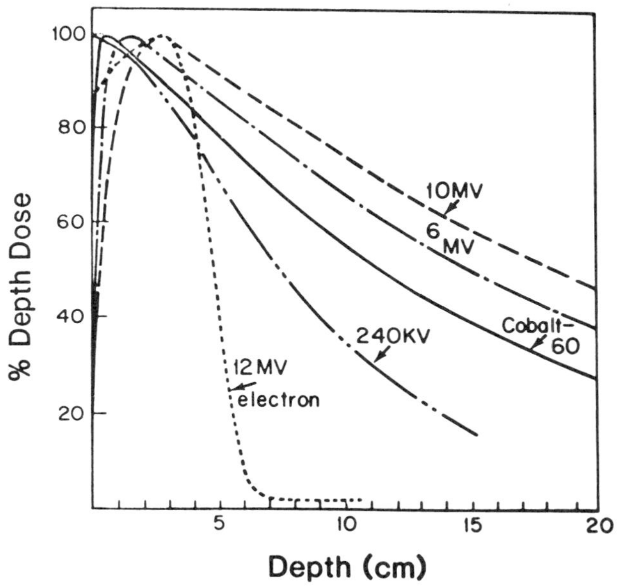

Figure 1.4. Depth dose characteristics for several selected radiation beams.

BRACHYTHERAPY

Interstitial Brachytherapy

Interstitial brachytherapy techniques involve implanting radioactive isotopes into a target volume. This results in the delivery of a high intensity of radiation within the volume. Interstitial implants can be either permanent or temporary. Permanently implanted radioisotopes usually have relatively short half-lives (days) or low radiation energies (HVL=cms of tissue) and therefore deliver a significant percentage of the dose within a short period of time or within a limited volume of tissue. Temporarily implanted radioisotopes have long half-lives (months to years) and high radiation energies (often >100 KeV) and are usually removed within several days of the implant to avoid overtreating normal tissue outside the implant or exposing the public to radiation. Radioisotopic material used for implant comes in several forms such as seeds, needles, wires and ribbons. Seeds can be individually implanted by means of specially designed injecting guns. Seeds also are placed in nylon ribbons which can be "threaded" into the tumor as described below.

Interstitial implants can be made by direct implantation of the radioisotope (preloading) or by use of an afterloading technique. With afterloading, hollow steel needles are inserted into the lesion. Plastic tubes are than placed inside the needles. The needles are subsequently removed leaving the plastic tubes in place in the lesion. Once a satisfactory implant arrangement is established, the radioactive isotope ribbon is threaded into the guiding hollow plastic tubes and secured in place with metal buttons at the ends of the tubes. This afterloaded insertion can be carried out rapidly and often is done in the patient's room; thus, sparing personnel from unnecessary exposure.

Typical isotopes used for permanent implants include Au-198 and I-125. Au-198 has a half-life of only 2.7 days. Therefore, 50% of the dose that will be given is given in the first 2.7 days. Less than two weeks following an implant (approximately five half-lives), Au-198 implants will have decayed to less than 5% of their activity at the time of implant. This short half-life makes Au 198 a useful radioisotope for permanent implants. Iodine-125 has a longer half-life (approximately 60 days) but emits lower energy radiation (25 KeV gamma, 21 KeV beta) which is rapidly absorbed by surrounding tissue (half value layer of 2 cm. of tissue). Thus, the low radiation energy of iodine-125 makes it an important radioisotope for permanent implants.

A typical temporary implanted isotope is Iridium -192. It emits gamma radiation of relatively high energy (300-612 KeV) with a half-life of 74 days. It can be directly applied to the target volume in the form of Iridium-192 wires and left in place for an amount of time necessary to give a previously specified dose to that volume. It can also be applied with an afterloading technique, usually in the form of ribbons.

Intracavitary Brachytherapy

Intracavitary brachytherapy is most frequently employed in gynecologic malignancies, particularly uterine and cervical carcinomas. Special hollow applicators are inserted into the uterine canal (a tandem applicator) and into the vaginal fornices (colpostats). After checking proper placement of the applicators with x-ray verification, the applicators are afterloaded with a radioisotope. Cesium-137 is an isotope used frequently in intracavitary insertions with a high energy (660 KeV) and long half-life (33 years). The insertion is, of course, temporary and precautions must be taken in limiting exposure (See Chapter 19). Cesium-137 has replaced radium-226 for use in intracavitary brachytherapy in most radiotherapy centers.

TREATMENT PLANNING

Radiotherapists seek to maximize dose absorbed by tumor and minimize dose delivered to normal tissue. Since tumors are frequently deep-seated or lie close to sensitive normal tissues, specialized treatment plans need to be devised. To achieve this, a treatment simulation or planning session, is undertaken prior to actual treatment initiation. During that session, technologists and dosimetrists aid the radiotherapist in establishing the treatment plan. Many variables need to be considered including the field size, number of treatment beams, beam direction and use of beam modifiers. Computerized dose distributions can be generated so that the therapist can choose the optimal treatment plan. Special alloy blocks can be custom made to block the beam from irradiating normal tissue. Wedge filters and tissue compensators sometimes are used to alter the radiation beam so that more uniform dose distribution can be obtained.

Proper immobilization and marking of the treatment fields are essential for consistent reproducibility in daily treatment. Lasers are used to check daily treatment position. Skin tattoos aid in lining up the treatment field. Casts made of plastic or other materials are occasionally constructed to conform to the patient's anatomy for proper immobilization.

REFERENCES

1. Johns HE and Cunningham JR: *The Physics of Radiology*. ed 3, Charles Thomas, NY, 1974.
2. Kramer S, Suntharalingam N, Zinninger G (ed): *High-energy Photons and Electrons: Clinical Applications in Cancer Management*. John Wiley & Sons, New York, NY 1976.

Chapter 2

Biology of Therapeutic Radiology

OVERVIEW

The biologic response of tumors and normal tissue to ionizing radiation is governed by a multitude of factors. The physical deposition of energy in living tissues through ionization initiates a chain of chemical reactions which results in cellular damage and ultimately in the observed clinical effect. It is at the cellular level that radiation biology has provided the most insight. Tissue and tumor response to radiation, though extensively studied, are very complex and presently can be only empirically described.

SUBCELLULAR RESPONSE TO RADIATION

Physical Factors

Ionizing radiation, whether electromagnetic or particulate, deposits energy through all parts of the cell unhindered by any intracellular barrier. The total energy absorbed per gram of tissue is quite small and relatively few molecules are ionized. For example, 400 rad results in an energy absorption of only about 10^{-3} calories per gram of tissue with only 1 of 50,000,000 molecules ionized. Although this dose appears to be sparsely ionizing, there are about 10^{22} molecules per gram of tissue so that more than 10^{15} molecules per gram will acquire enough energy to be ionized.

Ionization occurs along the paths of the high speed charged particles (e.g. electrons) that are set in motion by absorption of radiation energy. An important parameter describing the density of the ionization energy along these particle paths is the linear energy transfer (LET). It represents the amount of energy deposited in tissue per unit track length (KeV/). It is the physical parameter which accounts for the different biologic effectiveness of different types of radiation. Yet the concept of LET is relatively unimportant in clinical use, since the LET for most gamma and x-rays used in conventional radiotherapy varies only slightly with beam energies in use. Most high LET (densely ionizing) radiations, such as neutrons or alpha particles, are more efficient than gamma or X radiation and produce more biologic damage per rad dose. The relative biologic effectiveness (RBE) is a measure of the efficiency of radiation in producing a given biological response. By definition the RBE for a type of radiation (r) is given by:

$$RBE = D_{250}/D_r$$

where D250 and Dr are respectively the doses of 250 kv x-rays and of radiation (r) required to produce the same biologic response. The RBE, therefore, depends on (among other factors) the particular biologic response measured. The RBE for most conventional (low LET) gamma or X radiation is generally between 0.8 and 1.0. As LET increases, particularly between 10 and 100 KeV/ , so does RBE. Table 2.1 lists the approximate LET's and RBE's of several types of radiation.

Table 2.1
Approximate LET's and RBE's of several Types of Radiation.

Radiation Type	LET (KeV/)	RBE
Beta particle (1 MeV)	0.3	0.9
Cobalt-60	0.3	0.8-0.9
250KVP X-rays	2	1.0
Neutrons (19MeV)	0.5-15	1-2
Alpha Particles	30-100	5-10

Chemical Factors

Damage to critical molecules of the cell by radiation may result in important alterations in the biology of the cell. DNA is felt to be the most important target molecule. Damage to a target molecule may occur by direct effect of ionization of that molecule, or through an indirect effect, whereby the initial ionization occurs in a molecule other than the target, but the energy is subsequently transferred to the target molecule. The indirect effect is probably responsible for the majority of radiation damage. Water has been implicated as the mediator of the indirect effect through the formation of highly reactive free radicals and their diffusion to the target molecule. Chemical damage to DNA may take many forms, such as change or loss of a base, hydrogen bond breakage between strands, dimerization, crosslink formation and others. These can result in a change in molecular structure and function. Chromosome abnormalities are frequently observed post-radiation and are thought to be a major factor in cell killing.

The damage to molecules caused by radiation may be modified by a host of intracellular factors, including temperature, pH, oxygen concentration and target molecule concentration. Oxygen appears to be particularly important in determining radiation damage by modifying the number and type of free radicals produced. Radioprotective drugs can also modify radiation damage at this stage by chemically restoring (reducing) free radical damage to target molecules (See Chapter 20).

CELLULAR RESPONSE TO RADIATION

Pathologically, cells which have undergone radiation-induced cellular death are often swollen and vacuolated with loss of staining capacity, nuclear pyknosis and karyolysis. Giant cell production with cells growing to 25-200 times normal size may be seen. Degeneration and phagocytosis of these damaged cells usually ensues.

There are two major cellular effects observed following radiation: (1) loss of function and (2) loss of reproductive ability.

Loss of Function

Many non-dividing cells or cells with only a limited ability to divide undergo an interphase death with consequent loss of function. In nearly all non-dividing cells, such as adult nerve and muscle cells, interphase death occurs only after exposure to large doses of radiation (usually greater than 1000 rad). Lymphocytes, however, may undergo such a death after exposure to a much smaller radiation dose (less than 100 rad). Loss of function of single cells undergoing interphase death is not easily quantitated. The clinical importance of interphase death lies mostly in its contribution to death from whole body radiation (particularly due to lymphocyte death) and probably also in its contribution to late complications from high dose radiation.

Loss of Reproductive Ability

Loss of reproductive ability or "reproductive death" is the major effect of radiation on dividing cells. It signifies the loss of the cell's ability to produce viable progeny capable of sustained reproduction. Cell survival curves illustrate the dose-response relationship between a cell's ability to survive (resist a reproductive death) and radiation dose. Such survival curves have a general characteristic shape for most mammalian cells, whether tumor cells or normal cells (See Figure 2.1). The initial part or "shoulder" of the curve reflects the amount of damage that must be accumulated before lethal damage occurs. As the dose increases, the curve straightens to a line of constant slope (-1/Do) reflecting a direct logarithmic dose-response relationship. This relationship means that a given dose increment always results in the same fractional cell kill. The dose Do results in a fractional cell kill of (1-1/e) or 63% on this linear portion of the survival curve. Specific quantitative differences do exist in the survival curves between different cell lines. Cells with greater ability to accumulate or repair radiation damage have a survival curve with a larger shoulder. In the higher dose range the more radiosensitive the cell the steeper the slope.

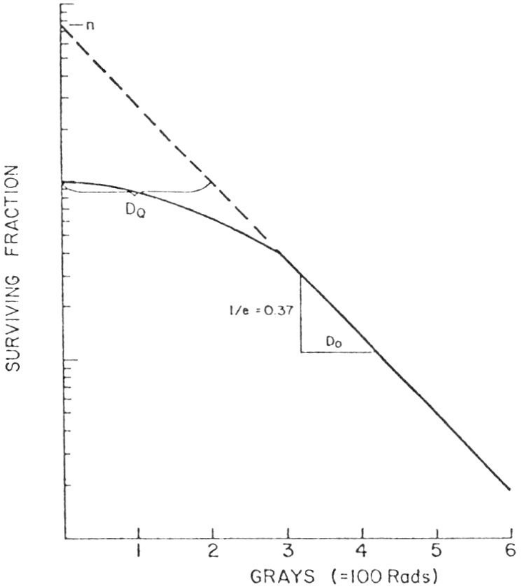

Figure 2.1. Idealized radiation survival curve (plotted on semi-log axes). Do is a measure of radiosensitivity on the straight line portion of the curve. Dq and n are measures of the curve (Dq = Do log n).

Several factors exist which may modify the radiation survival curve for a given cell line:

1. Oxygen: Oxygen aids in the production of damage by radiation-induced free radicals. Therefore, hypoxic and anoxic cells are relatively resistant to conventional (low LET) radiation. They exhibit survival curves with a broader shoulder and a less steep slope than well aerated cells. The ratio of doses required to produce the same survival in hypoxic compared to aerated cells is known as the oxygen enhancement ratio (OER) and equals approximately 3 for low LET radiation. High LET radiation is more efficient in producing damage and is less dependent on oxygen for its effect. Attempts at reducing the problem of relative radioresistance of hypoxic tumor cells include the use of "radiosensitizers" which mimic the effect of oxygen and

reduce the necessity for oxygen (See Chapter 20). During a course of radiation, tumors may reoxygenate as the tumor cell burden diminishes and oxygen becomes more readily available to remaining viable cells.

2. Repair of Sublethal Radiation Damage: Damage which can normally be repaired by the cell is known as sublethal damage. Sublethal damage is usually repaired within 2-6 hours following radiation. Sublethal damage by definition is not lethal but it does increase sensitivity to a subsequent irradiation. If a dose of radiation is followed by a second dose within a time period insufficient to allow adequate repair, the damage may be lethal. Exploitation of differences in repair capability in normal tissue and tumor tissue may be useful in developing more effective fractionation schemes (See Chapter 20).

3. Repair of Potentially Lethal Radiation Damage: Some damage which is lethal to a cell under normal growth conditions may be repaired under suboptimal or perturbed growth conditions. Such damage is referred to as potentially lethal damage (PLD). The relative importance of repair of such damage in clinical radiotherapy is not fully understood presently.

4. Dose Rate: When the dose rate diminishes, significantly more cells survive a given dose of radiation. This is due to the repair of sublethal damage during the radiation and to the proliferation of undamaged or still viable cells with very low dose rates. This effect is important in interstitial and intracavitary brachytherapy where dose rates are typically only 40 rad/hour compared to 100 rad/minute with external beam radiation. With the low dose rates used in brachytherapy a higher total dose can be given over a shorter overall of time due to repair and repopulation of normal tissues.

5. Cell Cycle Phase Dependence: Cell response to radiation is dependent on the phase of the cell cycle in which they are irradiated. Cells in mitosis (M) are most sensitive and cells in late nucleic acid synthesis (S) are least sensitive. The ratio of sensitivity between cells in M and cells in S may be 2.5 or more. Reassortment (or redistribution) of cells into sensitive

phases of the cell cycle could render them radiovulnerable. Unfortunately, such cell cycle dependence is difficult to exploit clinically since neither tumor cells nor tissues are easily synchronized in their cycling. Also, it is difficult to bring non-cycling cells into cycle.

TISSUE RESPONSE TO RADIATION

Radiation response of tissues represents a summation of the cellular effects both on tissue parenchymal cells and vascular stromal cells.

In tissues with a static population (called a non-renewable system) of non-dividing parenchymal cells, (for example neurons of the CNS and striated muscle cells), the critical damage of conventional fractionated radiation probably occurs in the vascular compartment, whereas the parenchymal cells of such tissues are relatively radioresistant. (Note: Increased capillary permeability can be seen with doses of less than 100 rad). Pathologically, acute damage is characterized by vascular dilatation, localized edema and inflammation. Chronic damage is seen as narrowing or occlusion of small vasculature with fibrosis and often a decrease in the number of parenchymal cells.

Tissues with dividing parenchymal cells under homeostatic control (called a renewal system) often sustain significant radiation damage to the parenchymal compartment as well as the vascular stromal compartment. In renewal systems cell equilibrium is normally present, since production of new cells is balanced by the death or migration of mature cells. A dose of radiation which kills most of the stem cells of the parenchymal compartment, will subsequently result in the depletion of functioning mature cells. Renewal systems with the shortest turnover times are affected earliest. Repopulation of stem cells and mature cells by remaining stem cells plays an important part in regaining tissue function postradiation. Table 2.2 indicates the approximate turnover time for selected renewal systems:

Table 2.2
Selected Renewal Systems and their approximate Turnover Time.

System	Turnover Time*
Blood	
RBC	120 days
Granulocyte	10 hours
Lymphocyte	Days to Years
G.I. Tract	
Oral Cavity	5 days
Stomach	3-9 days
Small Intestine	1.5 days
Colon	10 days
Skin	20 days
Respiratory Tract	
Tracheal Epithelium	50 days
Lung Alveolar Cells	10-30 days
Urinary Bladder	50 days
Testes	20 days
Eye	
Cornea	7 days

*Turnover Time: Time for replacement of number of cells equal to that in whole population.

ORGAN RESPONSE TO RADIATION

The tolerance of tissues and organs to radiation is an important clinical parameter. Generally, radiotherapists must limit the dose to a tumor to the tolerance dose of the surrounding normal tissues or organs. The minimum tolerance dose is defined as the TD5/5, that is the dose which will produce a given complication in no more than 5% of the patients in 5 years. The maximum tolerance dose (TD50/5) is the dose producing a 50% complication rate in 5 years. The tolerance dose depends on the type of fractionation used and volume of tissue irradiated.

Dose limiting organs have been separated into 3 classes based on their radiation tolerance. In Class I are organs in which radiation damage results in severe morbidity or mortality. In Class II are organs in which radiation damage results in mild to moderate morbidity (rarely mortality) and generally in late effects compatible with survival. Class III organs are those in which radiation damage results in either no morbidity or mild transient reversible effects. Table 2.3 list these organs along with their clinically reported tolerance doses (TD5/5 and TD50/5). Tolerance doses listed in Table 2.3 are based on <u>conventionally fractionated radiotherapy, i.e. single daily doses of 200 rad, 5 days per week</u>.

<u>Table 2.3a</u>
<u>Class I Organs</u> (from Rubin)

Class I Organs	Injury	$TD_{5/5}$	$TD_{50/5}$	Whole or Partial Organ (Field Size or Length)
Bone marrow	aplasia, pancytopenia	250	450	whole
		3000	4000	segmental
Liver	acute and chronic hepatitis	2500	4000	whole
		1500	2000	whole strip
Stomach	performation, ulcer hemorrhage	4500	5500	100 cm.^{2}
Intestine	ulcer, perforation, hemorrhage	4500	5500	400 cm.^{2}
		5000	6500	100 cm.^{2}
Brain	infarction, necrosis	6000	7000	whole
		7000	8000	25%
Spinal cord	infarction, necrosis	4500	5500	10 cm.
Heart	pericarditis and pancarditis	4500	5500	60%
Lung	acute and chronic pneumonitis	3000	3500	100 cm.^{2}
		1500	2500	whole
Kidney	acute and chronic nephrosclerosis	1500	2000	whole (strip)
		2000	2500	whole
Fetus	death	200	400	whole

Table 2.3b
Class II Organs (from Rubin)

Class III Organs	Injury	$TD_{5/5}$	$TD_{50/5}$
Muscle (child)	atrophy	2000-3000	4000-5000
Muscle (adult)	fibrosis	6000	8000
Lymph nodes and lymphatics	atrophy, sclerosis	5000	>7000
Large arteries and veins	sclerosis	>8000	>10,000
Articular cartilage	none	>50,000	>500,000
Uterus	necrosis, perforation	>10,000	>20,000
Vagina	ulcer, fistula	9000	>10,000
Breast (child)	no development	1000	1500
Breast (adult)	atrophy, necrosis	>5000	>10,000

Table 2.3c
Class III Organs

Class II Organs	Injury	$TD_{5/5}$	$TD_{50/5}$
Oral cavity and pharnyx	ulceration, mucositis	6000 —	7500
Skin	acute and chronic dermatitis	5500	7000
Esophagus	esophagitis, ulceration	6000	7500
Rectum	ulcer, stricture	6000	8000
Salivary glands	xerostomia	5000	7000
Bladder	contracture	6000	8000
Ureters	stricture	7500	10,000
Testes	sterilization	100	200
Ovary	sterilization	200-300	625-1200
Growing cartilage,	growth arrest,	1000	3000
bone (child)	dwarfting	1000	3000
Mature cartilage,	necrosis,	6000	10,000
bone (adult)	fracture, sclerosis	6000	10,000
Eye			
(a) Retina		5500	7000
(b) Cornea		5000	6000
(c) Lens		500	1200
Endocrine glands			
(a) Thyroid	hypothyroidism	4500	15,000
(b) Adrenal	hypoadrenalism	>6000	—
(c) Pituitary	hypopituitarism	4500	20,000-30,000
Peripheral nerves	neuritis	6000	10,000
Ear			
(a) Middle	Serous otitis	5000	7000
(b) Vestibular	Meniere's syndrome	6000	7000

TUMOR RESPONSE TO RADIATION

Tumor Eradication

The ability to eradicate a tumor is highly dependent on the size and radiosensitivity of the tumor. Repair, repopulation, reoxygenation and reassortment discussed earlier in the chapter (known as the four R's of radiobiology) play varying roles in tumor response to radiation. Many other factors, including tumor growth fraction and cell loss factor are also important.

Tumor size is obviously important in determing whether a tumor can be eradicated. Cell killing by radiation is an exponential function of the dose. Fewer fractions and a lower total dose are therefore required to eradicate microscopic disease (less than 10^6 cells) than for a 1 kilogram tumor (10^{12} cells). The radiation dose required for a given tumor control probability can be related to the tumor volume. The effect of size on tumor control is illustrated in Figure 2.2.

Tumor radiosensitivity: There is a wide range of radiosensitivity to conventional radiation doses among tumors. Among the most sensitive are the leukemias, lymphomas, seminomas and dysgerminomas. Among the least sensitive are the melanomas and sarcomas. (Note that radiosensitivity and radioresistance are relative terms and that given a high enough dose large numbers of even "radioresistant" cells can be killed by radiation.) The effect of radiosensitivity on tumor control is also illustrated in Figure 2.2.

Reoxygenation is the only one of the "4 R's" which occurs in tumors but not in normal tissues. Normal tissues contain no or few hypoxic cells, whereas tumors may contain 5-20% hypoxic cells due to the limited diffusion distance of oxygen (about 180 microns) from an often inadequate tumor vascular supply. The extent to which tumors reoxygenate during a course of radiation may help determine whether they can be eradicated by radiation.

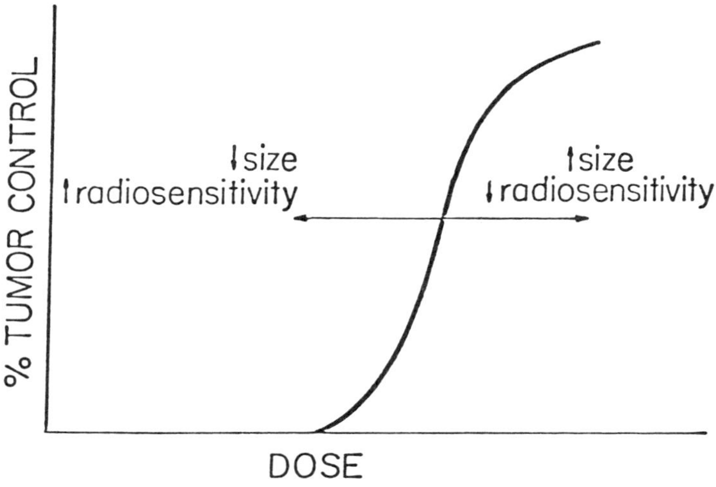

Figure 2.2. Sigmoid curve of tumor control as a function of dose. Differences in tumor size and radiosensitivity may shift the curve to the right or left as illustrated.

Tumor Radiocurability

The radiocurability of tumors depends not only on the radiosensitivity of the tumor but also on the normal tissue tolerance. The therapeutic ratio is a measure of radiocurability and is described by the following relationship:

$$TR = \frac{\text{normal tissue tolerance dose}}{\text{tumor lethal dose}}$$

where normal tissue tolerance and tumor lethal dose must be individually defined for the specific tumor and tissue in question. The goal of curative (definitive) radiotherapy is to produce local tumor eradication without unacceptable complications. The radiotherapist tries to use a dose of radiation which will maximize tumor control and minimize (or keep within "acceptable limits") the risk of significant complications as illustrated in Figure 2.3.

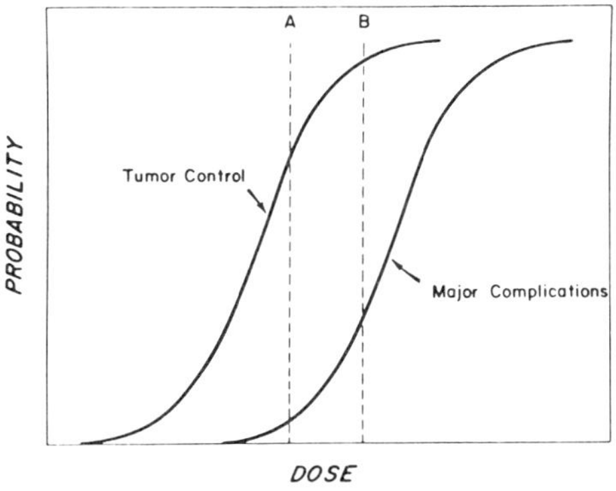

Figure 2.3 (from DeVita)
Sigmoid curves of tumor control and complications.
A, Dose for tumor control with minimum complications.
B, Maximum tumor control with significant complications.

RESPONSE TO WHOLE BODY RADIATION

Whole body exposures to radiation give rise to 3 major dose-dependent syndromes: the hematopoietic, gastrointestinal and central nervous system syndromes. An outline of the clinically important aspects of these syndromes is presented in Table 2.4.

The treatment of patients exposed to whole body radiation depends on the dose received. At doses of a few hundred rad, death is caused by damage to the hematopoietic system. In man this occurs 30 to 60 days after the radiation exposure. The dose causing 50% mortality within 60 days from the radiation is known as the LD 50/60 and is about 400 rad in man. Patients receiving over 700 rad will die regardless of treatment. All those receiving under 200 rad should survive with few, if any, symptoms. Treatment is believed to be effective in reducing fatalities in patients receiving doses within 200-600 rad.

Table 2.4
Whole Body Radiation Syndromes - CNS, GI, and Hematopoietic - following single acute exposure to radiation

	CNS Syndrome	G.I. Syndrome	Hematopoietic Syndrome
Target Organ	Brain	Small Bowel	Bone Marrow
Threshold dose (symptoms)	2000	500	150
Threshold dose (death)	?5000	1000	250
LD_{50}*	?10,000	?2000	400
Latent Period	Minutes to Hours	3-5 days	2-3 weeks
Death	First 2 days	2 days-2 weeks	3-6 weeks
Symptoms (Clinical)	Confusion ataxia coma convulsion	Malaise anorexia nausea vomiting diarrhea dehydration	Malaise fever purpura infection
Major Pathology	vasculitis encephalitis meningitis edema	depletion of intestinal epithelium	Bone Marrow hypocellularity

*where LD_{50} is the dose resulting in 50% mortality.

The principal cause of death in patients who can be helped by treatment is infection. Patients should be hospitalized and isolated. Cultures and sensitivities from accessible sites should be obtained. Hematologic parameters should be followed closely. Clinical infections require vigorous antibiotic treatment. Hemorrhages should be treated with red cell replacement and platelet transfusion. Nutrition must be maintained and fluids and electrolytes replaced as needed. The value of bone marrow transplant in aplastic individuals is controversial. The genetic and carcinogenic effects of whole body radiation are discussed in Chapter 19.

REFERENCES

1. Hall E: Radiobiology for the Radiologist 2nd ed Harper and Row, Hagerstown, MD, 1978.
2. Ritter M: The radiobiology of mammalian cells. Semin Oncol 8:3-17, 1981.
3. Rubin P and Cassarett GW: Clinical Radiation Pathology, vol I, II. WB Saunders, Philadelphia PA, 1968.
4. Rubin P, Cooper R and Philips TL (eds): Radiation Biology and Radiation Pathology Syllabus (SHRT 1: Radiation Oncology). American College of Radiology, Chicago, 1975.
5. DeVita V, Hellman S, Rosenberg S: chpt 7, Cancer - Principles and Practice of Oncology, Principles of Radiation Therapy, p 118, Lippincott Co, Philadelphia, PA, 1982.

Chapter 3

Skin Cancer and Melanoma

NON-MELANOMA SKIN CANCER

OVERVIEW

Malignancies of the skin are common with a yearly incidence of approximately 310,000 cases. On the basis of differing biologic behaviors, it is imperative to consider melanomas and non-melanoma skin cancers separately. Non-melanoma skin cancer, such as basal cell and squamous cell carcinomas, occasionally metastasize but then only late in the course of the disease. On the other hand, even relatively small primary melanomas tend to disseminate to regional lymphatics and distant sites.

There is a tendency for clinicians to take non-melanoma skin cancers lightly since cure rates are quite excellent. The question arises whether there is a difference between the biologic behavior of a non-melanoma skin cancer and a typical squamous cell carcinoma of the lung. Part of the answer probably lies in the _volume_ of tumor present in each situation. Superficial skin malignancies are readily detectable and treated quite early. On the contrary, bronchogenic carcinomas often grow to rather large volumes before producing symptoms. If the same volume of cancer contained in a typical, fist-sized lung lesion were to be flattened out into a 2 or 3 mm thick sheet, it would cover most of the anterior chest wall. Even skin malignancies of this size are rarely curable, having disseminated widely.

PATHOLOGY & CLINICAL FEATURES

BASAL CELL CARCINOMA

Basal cell carcinomas, also called basal cell epitheliomas, tend to spread by direct extension, although lymphatic involvement is seen on rare occasions. Microscopically, these tumors arise from the pluripotential basal cells of the epidermis. They may grow in sheets with microscopic cords invading deeply along nerves, fascial planes and vessels. Clinically, they vary in size from millimeters to centimeters and usually have raised, pearly borders with central umbilication. Ulceration, crusting and telangiectasia may also be present. If neglected, they can grow to a large size with destruction of much of the face presenting as the classic "rodent ulcer". Etiologic factors in the development of these malignancies include sunlight and x-ray exposure.

SQUAMOUS CELL CARCINOMA

Squamous cell carcinomas of the skin are somewhat more aggressive than basal cell carcinomas. Predisposing factors include senile keratosis, leukoplakia, arsenical keratosis, burn scarring, actinic keratosis and radiodermatitis. Microscopically, they may vary in differentiation from low grade with keratin pearl formation to high grade anaplastic lesions. If the basal layer is still intact, intraepidermal squamous cell carcinoma or Bowen's disease is present. Bowen's disease, often confused with eczema, may be associated with an internal malignancy in 25% of affected patients. Erythroplasia of Queyrat is a term for intradermal squamous cell carcinoma involving the glans penis or the vulva and represents a malignant condition.

OTHER SKIN MALIGNANCIES

Other malignancies of the skin and its appendages include subungual carcinomas, sweat gland carcinoma and sebaceous gland adenocarcinoma.

Mycosis fungoides, a T-cell lymphoma of multicentric origin, initially involves the skin and when associated with circulating malignant cells is termed Sezary syndrome. Microscopically, this is characterized by atypical histiocytic skin infiltrates called Pautrier's microabscesses. This lymphoma involves skin primarily and lymph nodes and viscera secondarily in distinction from other non-Hodgkin's lymphomas. Three classical cutaneous stages are described: (1) premycotic or eczematous stage, (2) infiltrative, plaque stage and (3) tumoral stage.

Kaposi's sarcoma is a malignancy showing endothelial and fibroblastic proliferation with formation of new thin-walled blood vessels. Often there is hemorrhage and inflammatory response. Multiple blue-red to brownish nodules and plaques are seen on the skin. This cutaneous malignancy is usually found in elderly males of Mediterranian extraction such as Jews and Italians. In recent years Kaposi's sarcoma has been reported in patients suffering from acquired immunodeficiency syndrome (*AIDS*). In this group of patients the *lymphadenopathic* form is more common and the disease is biologically more aggressive. Other presentations include the *nodular*, *florid* and *infiltrative* types.

STAGING

A TNM staging system has been proposed for non-melanoma skin cancers. However, this is not in wide clinical use.

WORK-UP

During history taking, attention should be paid to exposure to *arsenicals* such as Fowler's solution and other known skin carcinogens such as *methylchloranthanrene*, *benzpyrene* and tars. Sun exposure and prior radiotherapy for conditions such as acne, tinea capitis or thymic enlargement should also be noted. Patients of Celtic origin are at risk for developing skin malignancies in sun-damaged skin. Blacks have a low incidence.

During the physical exam, the surface characteristics and pigmentation of the lesion should be described. An attempt should be made to estimate the depth and peripheral extension of the skin lesions. Mohs has shown that tumor cords may extend for 1-2 cm into the surrounding tissue beyond the visible and palpable extent of the lesion. This fact must be kept in mind in planning a surgical or radiotherapeutic approach. In the case of squamous cell carcinomas, regional lymph nodes deserve special attention.

All suspicious skin lesions should be biopsied. Small lesions may be removed by excisional biopsy if the location will permit. The pathologist must examine all margins including the deep margin of resection. For larger lesions or any location where excisional biopsy would leave an unacceptable cosmetic defect, an incisional or punch biopsy can be obtained. For patients with multiple keratoses, frequent petroleum jelly applications can be recommended for a one month period. If the lesions persist, biopsy should be carried out.

TREATMENT AND RESULTS

Several factors must be considered in planning the treatment of any skin cancer for which there are several equally effective treatment modalities.

1. Size
2. Location
3. Age of patient
4. Patient convenience

Local excision or electrocautery following a biopsy is often curative for basal and squamous cell cancers. These procedures have the advantage of providing a rapid cure with no late effects to the surrounding normal tissue.

Radiotherapy yields a high cure rate. When the nasal tip or alae, the pinna, eyelids or canthi are involved, surgery may yield unacceptable cosmetic results. Tumors located in the perinasal folds or in the inner canthi of the eyelids often display microscopic extension of tumor far exceeding the grossly observed or palpated margins. In these situations radiotherapy has a special role.

The dose of radiation required to control skin carcinoma will result in a moderate moist desquamation. The patient should be advised of this at the start of treatment, although the peak reaction often occurs several days following completion of therapy. In general, a more highly fractionated course of radiotherapy yields a superior cosmetic result; however, this must be balanced against the need for expediency. Also, the volume of tissue to be irradiated will influence the choice of a daily dose; thus, larger areas of skin will display more severe acute and late reactions when higher daily fractions are chosen. Typical treatment schemes may vary from a dose of 5000 rad in 10 equal treatments over two weeks to 4800 rad in 16 fractions over three and a half weeks to 7000 rad over an eight week period. The choice will depend on tumor location, size, previous treatment and the desired cosmetic result.

The depth to which the lesion must be treated will influence the choice of the quality of radiation. Superficial or orthovoltage equipment is adequate, producing 100 to 250 KeV radiations. Aluminum or copper filters of appropriate thickness will modify the quality of these beams and the percent depth dose. In recent years linear accelerators or betatrons capable of producing electron beams with energies varying from 2 to 10 MeV have become widely available, and may be used to irradiate a superficial slab of tissue. Other treatment options include the use of surface plaques or applicators through which iridium-192 or radium needles are placed using well-defined rules of distribution.

Mohs' chemosurgery, during which the extent of excision is monitored by carefully mapping the tumor and assessing the margins of resection with a frozen section technique, is particularly effective in the case of recurrent tumors. This is time consuming and requires the availability of an expert dermatopathologist. It may be done using fresh tissue or zinc chloride fixed tissue.

The topical application of 5-fluorouracil has been used for the treatment of premalignant actinic keratoses but must be considered investigational in the treatment of proven skin carcinoma. Immunotherapy using 2-4 dinitrochlorobenzene (DNCB) has also been used experimentally for the treatment of multiple skin cancers in patients with x-ray dermatitis, xeroderma pigmentosa and arsenical keratoses. It probably has no role in the routine treatment of the above mentioned skin malignancies.

Surgery is the preferred treatment for burn carcinomas, which also have a high incidence of regional metastases. Since the underlying scar tissue would be less well vascularized, theoretically, tumor hypoxia would make these tumors relatively radioresistant. Because of their rarity, there is scant literature to support the optimal management of subungual carcinomas, sweat gland carcinomas and sebaceous gland carcinomas. Traditionally, these have been handled surgically, although radiation therapy has been applied to advanced inoperable or recurrent tumors with predictably disappointing results.

No matter what modalities are employed in the treatment of basal cell carcinomas, cure rates of 90-95% are obtained. For squamous cell carcinomas, 75-85% of patients are cured. For burn scar carcinomas, five-year survival rates vary from 31% for lower extremity lesions to 51% for head and neck lesions. Subungual carcinomas treated by amputation have yielded a five-year actuarial survival rate of 100%. A five-year survival rate for sweat gland carcinomas in one series was 50% but the disease-free survival was only 38%. The prognosis in this disorder seems to be related to lymph node involvement. Sebaceous gland carcinomas of the skin carry a good prognosis with an 80% cure rate.

Mycosis Fungoides: Formerly, therapy for mycosis fungoides was considered strictly palliative and aggressive measures were felt to be unwarranted in the early stages. Treatments such as topical steroids with and without occlusive dressings, oral psoralens photochemotherapy, topical mechlorethamine and topical nitrosoureas have been shown to ameliorate the signs and symptoms of the disease. Experience at some 30 medical centers throughout the United States and Canada has demonstrated the usefulness of total-skin electron beam therapy. Using specially modified low energy linear accelerators to produce electron beams of 2.5-4.0 MeV, the whole body surface area is treated to doses ranging from 2400 rad to 3600 rad over a 3 to 9 week period. This therapy will induce complete remissions in 70-85% of patients in the earlier stages of the disease with many patients experiencing prolonged disease-free survival. A dose response relationship has been documented by the Stanford experience with a complete remission rate of 90% for patients receiving over 3000 rad and a complete remission of only 18% for patients receiving less than 1000 rad. Recurrence following total skin electron irradiation may be related to areas of underdosing in the skin fold and subcutaneous tissue as well as receding of the skin from circulating neoplastic T-cells. The side effects from this therapy include temporary hair loss, onycholysis, increased skin erythema, hyperpigmentation and late skin atrophy. Because the range of electrons of this energy is only 10 to 20 mm, no hematologic toxicity has been observed. In patients who have unresponsive skin disease or manifest visceral involvement, systemic chemotherapy has been of benefit. Active agents include mechlorethamine, cyclophosphamide, actinomycin-D, streptonigrin, high-dose methotrexate with citrovorum rescue and thymidine infusions.

Kaposi's sarcoma is quite radiosensitive and when localized it can be controlled with relatively small doses of radiation. Some authors recommend single doses from 800 to 1000 rad using generous fields, while others prefer fractionated irradiation delivering 2500 rad over a two and a half week period. Cobalt teletherapy or megavoltage beams are often used in the treatment of Kaposi's sarcoma since the subcutaneous tissues may be involved. Quite often the skin lesions are associated with lymphedema of the extremities, which will respond slowly to treatment using these more penetrating radiations. When Kaposi's sarcoma recurs locally following multiple courses of irradiation or disseminates distantly, chemotherapy can produce remissions. Active agents include actinomycin-D, vinca alkaloids and DTIC.

MORBIDITY OF SKIN IRRADIATION

Acute

Acute reactions include erythema, which may appear as soon as 24 hours after treatment depending on the quality or skin-sparing properties of the beam and the fraction size. The onset, duration and intensity of this reaction are dose-dependent. Depending on the total dose, erythema will be followed by a dry desquamation. If all cells of the basal layer are killed, these cells will be completely shed exposing the dermis and causing serous fluid to weep from the surface, i.e., a moist desquamation. Repopulation of the dermis will than occur from the edges of the field and from the epithelial cells of the hair follicles, which are more resistant than the basal cell layer. Fowler and associates proposed a grading system for the degree of radiation reaction in pig skin, and this has been adopted with modifications for work in the clinic (See Table 3.1). Necrosis can be seen as a severe acute reaction.

Table 3.1
Skin Reaction:Fowler Scale

Arbitary score	Reaction
0	No visible reaction
1	Faint erythema
2	Erythema
3	Marked erythema
4	Moist desquamation of less than half the irradiated area
5	Moist desquamation of more than half the irradiated area

Treatment of acute radiation reactions should be directed towards maintaining an intact epithelium; therefore, any physical trauma no matter how slight should be minimized. The patient should be instructed not to scratch or rub the skin in the irradiated fields. Often times, scratching will occur during sleep and a patient may need to wear a pair of mittens to protect the skin. The skin may be washed with a mild soap; however, scrubbing is prohibited. After the soap is rinsed off, the skin should be patted dry, not rubbed. Loose cotton underwear as well as soft cotton clothing over the treated area is preferred. The patient should not use lotions, perfumes or astringents in the treated area without permission of the radiation therapist. When a moist reaction is evident, the affected area should be cleansed with dilute hydrogen peroxide solution. A 1% aqueous gentian violet solution may then be applied to the area of moist desquamation. If infection is evident, an antibiotic ointment may be used. Some therapists recommend the application of corticosteroid creams to prevent dusky erythema from progressing to a moist desquamation. This will often relieve pruritus as will the application of cornstarch.

Late Reaction

Hyperpigmentation, hypopigmentation, telangiectasia and skin atrophy are late effects. Permanent epilation is also a frequent late effect and is dose dependent. Subcutaneous fibrosis with woody induration of the tissues can also be seen in fields receiving a high dose using skin-sparing megavoltage radiations. Necrosis secondary to trauma, burns or frostbite are also possible.

MELANOMA

OVERVIEW

Melanomas are malignant tumors of ectodermal origin arising from the melanocyte. Embryologically, this cell is derived from neural crest cells and may be found in skin, eye (choroid and ciliary body) and other sites such as the upper respiratory tract, gastrointestinal tract, bladder and reproductive system.

PATHOLOGY & CLINICAL FEATURES

At the present time it is believed that most melanomas arise de novo but with up to 30% arising in pre-existent nevi. Pathologically, the differential diagnosis includes an active junctional nevus, juvenile melanoma and pigmented basal cell carcinoma. Three types of melanoma are described:

1. Superficial spreading melanoma
2. Lentigo maligna melanoma
3. Nodular melanoma

Lentigo maligna melanoma typically presents in elderly individuals with a median age of 70. They account for 10% of melanomas and tends to grow horizontally in a plaque-like manner. Superficial spreading and nodular melanomas account for 60% and 30% of melanomas, respectively. The median age for both is approximately 50 years. As the name implies, superficial spreading melanomas grow horizontally but they do have a raised palpable component. Nodular melanomas tend to display vertical growth.

Pathologists have made significant contributions to the management of malignant melanoma. In 1965 Clark described five levels of invasion, which have been correlated with the propensity for lymph node metastases and subsequent survival (See Table 3.2).

Table 3.2
Clark's Histologic Staging

Level	Extent of Inavsion
I	In situ, confined to the epidermis
II	Invading the papillary zone of the dermis, with perhaps a few cells down to the reticular dermis
III	Cells accumulating along the interface of the papillary and reticular layers, wihtout invasion of the reticular dermis
IV	Invasion of the reticular zone of the dermis
V	Invasion of subcutaneous fat

Likewise, the measured thickness of a lesion has been shown by Breslow to be of prognostic significance. Table 3.3 depicts the correlation between the incidence of lymph node metastases and the corresponding Clark's level and also the thickness of the primary lesion.

Table 3.3
Incidence of Regional Node Metastases

Clark's Level	% Nodal Metastases	Breslow Thickness (in mm)
I - II	0 - 5%	< 0.76
III	15%	0.76 - 1.5
IV	35%	1.5 - 4
V	50%	> 4

As with non-melanotic cancers, sun exposure and Celtic ancestry seem to be related to the epidemiology of this disease. Other prognostic factors include the patient's age and sex.

STAGING

A TNM Classification exists which incorporates both Clark's level and lesion thickness.

TNM Classification

Primary Tumor (T)

- TX No evidence of primary tumor (unknown primary or primary tumor removed and not histologically examined)
- T0 Atypical melanocytic hyperplasia (Clark Level I); not a malignant lesion
- T1 Invasion of papillary dermis (Level II) or 0.78 mm thickness or less
- T2 Invasion of the papillary-reticular-dermal interface (Level III) or 0.76 to 1.5 mm thickness
- T3 Invasion of the reticular dermis (Level IV) or 1.5 to 4.0 mm thickness
- T4 Invasion of subcutaneous tissue (Level V) or 4.1 mm or greater thickness, or satellite(s) within 2 cm of any primary melanoma

Nodal Involvement (N)

- NX Minimum requirements to assess the regional nodes cannot be met.
- N1 Involvement of only one regional lymph node station; node(s) movable and not over 5 cm in diameter, or negative regional lymph nodes and the presence of less than five in-transit metastases beyond 2 cm from the primary site
- N2 Any one of the following: (1) involvement of more than one regional lymph node station; (2) regional node(s) over 5 cm in diameter or fixed; (3) five or more in-transit metastases or any in-transit metastases beyond 2 cm from the primary site with regional lymph node involvement

Distant Metastasis (M)

- MX Not assessed
- M0 No known distant metastasis
- M1 Involvement of skin or subcutaneous tissue beyond the site of primary lymph node drainage

Staging Group

Stage IA	T1, N0, M0
Stage IB	T2, N0, M0
Stage IIA	T3, N0, M0
Stage IIB	T4, N0, M0
Stage III	Any T, N1, M0
Stage IV	Any T, any N, M1 or M2

WORK-UP

Note should be made of any history of change in the size, thickness or color of a skin lesion. Melanomas are often pruritic, friable and bleed easily.

Ulceration of cutaneous melanomas has proved to be an adverse finding. A history of any prior dermal surgical procedures and whether or not histologic studies were obtained should be sought. The physical characteristics of the skin lesion such as margins, color, size and the presence of satellite lesions should be recorded. Assessment of regional lymph nodes is mandatory. Since distant metastases are not uncommon, an evaluation of liver, lungs and central nervous system should be carried out.

As with skin cancers, biopsy of suspicious pigmented lesions is essential. Smaller lesions may be removed by excisional biopsy, with punch biopsy being reserved for larger tumors. The importance of microstaging has been stated. Electron microscopy can be performed to look for granules in amelanotic lesions. On the basis of the prognostic characteristics of the primary tumor, a search for distant metastases can be made. All patients should have chest x-rays and blood chemistries. Radionuclide scans of liver, brain and bone can be reserved for patients with a high likelihood for dissemination.

TREATMENT

MANAGEMENT OF THE PRIMARY LESION

Traditionally, the primary tumor had been managed surgically using wide local excision with skin grafting. Five centimeter margins are advocated by some authors while others believe 3 cm is adequate. These policies result in local recurrence in less than 5% of patients. Grafts are required to provide skin coverage. Radiotherapy has been used as definitive treatment for primary cutaneous melanomas, although historically these tumors are considered radioresistant. Many of the early series using radiotherapy as primary treatment have included a high proportion of unbiopsied lesions, making the results suspect since pigmented basal cell carcinomas can masquerade as melanomas. There are, however, reports of the use of radiotherapy in the treatment of lentigo maligna melanoma as an alternative to surgical excision. Recently, conservative excision followed by postoperative irradiation has been advanced as an acceptable alternative to wide local excision, which often yields a poor cosmetic result.

MANAGEMENT OF REGIONAL LYMPHATICS

The incidence of lymph node metastases increases dramatically with increasing thickness of the primary lesion and increasing extent of invasion by Clark's Level (See Table 3.3). The role of prophylactic lymph node dissection for clinical stage I melanoma remains controversial. When the regional nodes are clinically involved, therapeutic lymphadenectomy is indicated. Radiotherapy has no proven value in the management of nodal metastases.

ADJUVANT CHEMOTHERAPY

Prevention of distant metastatic disease in high risk patients with thick or locally invasive primary lesions or with regional lymph node involvement has been the rationale for combining surgery with adjuvant chemotherapy or immunotherapy. Such adjuvant treatment has not yet resulted in significant survival improvement.

RADIOTHERAPY

Cutaneous melanomas have been considered relatively radioresistant. This dictum has been challenged by several investigators. There is radiobiologic evidence that in vitro melanoma cell lines demonstrate a large shoulder on the radiation dose response curve. Although this is disputed by some researchers, it is the rationale for the use of large fraction radiotherapy in the treatment of melanoma with fraction sizes varying from 400 to 800 rad. On the basis of retrospective studies, some authors claim significant local control rates using conventional fractions of 200 to 300 rad as long as the total dose is greater than 4000 rad. It is likely that the present controversy can only be settled by a prospective randomized clinical trial such as the one currently being conducted by ECOG. The reputed value of large fraction irradiation has been demonstrated for skin, lymph node metastases, intra-thoracic and visceral metastases but not for bone and central nervous system metastases.

MANAGEMENT OF METASTATIC MELANOMA

Systemic chemotherapy has not dramatically impacted upon the survival of patients with metastatic melanoma. DTIC is one of the most active agents with a response rate of approximately 20%. Nitrousoureas are also active with a rate of 15%. Dibromodulcitol as a single agent has activity reported as high as 25%. Combinations of bleomycin, vinblastine, and DTIC and BCNU, vincristine and DTIC have yielded response rates ranging from 20-30%. Non-specific immunotherapy has not significantly improved these results, although intralesional injection of BCG can cause regression of injected skin metastases and some non-injected lesions but have no effect on visceral disease.

RESULTS

The prognosis of melanomas is dependent upon the level of invasion and thickness of the primary lesion. The five-year survival for patients with Level II melanomas is approximately 85%; for Level III, 68%; for Level IV, 50% and for Level V, 21%. Regional lymph node metastases carry a grave prognosis. The overall survival for node negative patients is approximately 72% falling to 29% where there is nodal involvement. For patients presenting with distant metastases from malignant melanoma, the median survival is approximately five months.

NON-CUTANEOUS MELANOMA

Because of their rarity, the optimal treatment of non-cutaneous melanoma has not been defined. Harwood et al have reported the Princess Margaret Hospital experience with radiation therapy for melanomas arising from the mucosal surfaces in the head and neck. Complete local control was maintained in 11 of 24 patients; again the efficacy of fraction sizes of 400 rad or greater was suggested. The prognosis for all but the thinnest melanomas in the anorectal region is quite poor with a 12% survival rate at Memorial Sloan-Kettering Cancer Center following radical surgery. The management of ocular melanoma will be discussed in Chapter 6.

REFERENCES

1. Freitag SB, Culmane DL: Neoplasms of the skin and malignant melanoma. Chicago, Year Book, 1976.
2. von Essen CF: Roentgen therapy of skin and lip carcinoma: factors influencing success and failure. Am J Roentgen 83:556-570, 1960.
3. Mohs FE: Chemosurgery, Microscopically Controlled Surgery for Skin Cancer. Charles C. Thomas, pp 3-18, Springfield, IL, 1978.
4. Tadros AAM et al: Total skin electron irradiation for mycosis fungoides: failure analysis and prognostic factors. I J Rad Onc Bio Phys 9:1279-1287.
5. Overgaard J: Radiation treatment of malignant melanoma. I J Rad Onc Bio Phys 6:41-44, 1981.
6. Katz HR: The results of different fractionation schemes in the palliative irradiation of metastatic melanoma. I J Rad Onc Bio Phys 7:907-911, 1981.

Chapter 4

Head and Neck Cancer

OVERVIEW

Patients with cancer of head and neck regions require a multidisciplinary approach in management. The initial assessment and treatment decision are crucial since salvage therapy for local recurrence in many head and neck sites is frequently unsuccessful and recurrences often are associated with disseminated disease. The nutritional status of these patients is often poor due to the tumor, and many patients have a history of heavy usage of both alcohol and cigarettes. Overall, these patients represent difficult management problems.

PATHOLOGY

Most cancers of the head and neck arise from mucosal surfaces and are squamous cell carcinomas or variants including lymphoepithelioma, spindle cell carcinoma, verrucous carcinoma and undifferentiated carcinoma. Adenocarcinomas are found in glandular sites (salivary, thyroid, lacrimal) or may be metastatic to the head or neck. Lymphomas, solitary plasmacytomas, and sarcomas are also encountered (these tumors are covered in other chapters).

CLINICAL FEATURES

Head and neck cancers show a male predominance and occur most frequently in the 50-60 year age group. There is usually a history of heavy cigarette and/or alcohol usage. Second primary lesions of the upper aerodigestive tract are seen in 15-20% of patients.

These malignancies can present as fungating exophytic masses, invasive endophytic ulcerations or verrucous growths. Endophytic lesions often have ill-defined borders and are aggressive and difficult to control compared to exophytic growths.

Presenting symptoms depend on location, (a mass in the neck may be seen with <u>any</u> of these lesions):

Oral cavity - pain, swelling, ulceration, trismus (invasion of masticatory muscles)
Oropharynx - dysphagia, local pain or referred otalgia
Hypopharynx - dysphagia, weight loss, hoarseness
Larynx - hoarseness, local pain, dysphgia, dyspnea
Nose/Paranasal Sinuses - local pain, bleeding, obstuction to breathing
Nasopharynx - nasal obstruction, epistaxis, otitis media, cranial nerve deficits

STAGING

<u>Primary Sites</u> (T Categories)

<u>Oral Cavity</u>:

TIS:	Carcinoma in situ
T1:	Tumor 2 cm. or less
T2:	Tumor 2-4 cm.
T3:	Tumor > 4 cm.
T4:	Massive tumor > 4 cm. with deep invasion of antrum, pterygoid muscles, root of tongue, or skin of neck

<u>Supraglottic Larynx</u>:

TIS:	Carcinoma in situ
T1:	Tumor confined to site of origin with normal mobility
T2:	Tumor extension to adjacent supraglottic sites or glottis without fixation
T3:	Tumor limited to larynx with fixation and/or extension to postcricoid area, medial wall of pyriform sinus, or pre-epiglottic space
T4:	Massive tumor extending beyond the larynx to involve oropharynx, soft tissues of neck, or destruction of thyroid cartilage

<u>Glottic Larynx</u>:

TIS:	Carcinoma in situ
T1:	Tumor confined to vocal cords with normal mobility
T2:	Supraglottic and/or subglottic tumor extension with normal or impaired vocal cord mobility

T3: Tumor confined to larynx with vocal cord fixation

T4: Massive tumor with thyroid cartilage destruction and/or extension beyond confines of larynx

Paranasal Sinuses:

T0: No evidence of primary tumor

T1: Tumor confined to antral mucosa without bone erosion or destruction

T2: Tumor confined to suprastructure mucosa without bone destruction, or to infrastructure with destruction of medial or inferior bony walls only

T3: Extensive tumor invading skin or cheek, orbit, anterior ethmoid sinuses, or pterygoid muscle

T4: Massive tumor with invasion of pterygoid plate, posterior ethmoids, nasopharynx, pterygoid plates, or base of skull

Nasopharynx:

TIS: Carcinoma in situ

T1: Tumor confined to one nasopharyngeal site or no tumor visible (biopsy positive)

T2: Tumor involving two nasopharyngeal sites

T3: Tumor extension into nasal cavity or oropharynx

T4: Skull invasion, cranial nerve involvement, or both

Oropharynx:

TIS: Carcinoma in situ

T1: Tumor 2 cm. or less

T2: Tumor 2-4 cm.

T3: Tumor > 4 cm.

T4: Massive tumor with invasion of bone, soft tissues of neck, or root of tongue

Cervical Lymph Nodes (applicable to all head and neck sites)

N0: Nodes clinically univolved

N1: Single clinically positive homolateral node < 3 cm.

N2a: Single clinically positive homolateral node 3-6 cm.

N2b: Multiple clinically positive homolateral nodes, all < 6 cm.

N3a: Clinically positive homolateral node(s), at least one > 6 cm.
N3b: Bilateral clinically positive nodes
N3c: Contralateral clinically positive nodes only

Stage Grouping:

Stage I:	T1, N0, M0
Stage II:	T2, N0, M0
Stage III:	T3, N0, M0
	T1,2,3; N1, M0
Stage IV:	T4, N0, N1, M0
	any T1, N2,3; M0
	any T1, any N, M1

WORK-UP

Physical exam with mapping of primary tumor and neck node involvement (See Figure 4.1). Biopsy of primary, if no primary then biopsy of neck node (see below regarding biopsy of neck nodes). Indirect mirror exam and endoscopy. Radiologic studies: chest x-ray is always needed and bone scan, panorex of the mandible, tomograms or CT scan of specific sites may also be needed. Chemistries: CBC, liver studies, SMA-12 (see specific sites for details). Epstein-Barr virus titres may be elevated in lymphoepitheliomas of the nasopharynx.

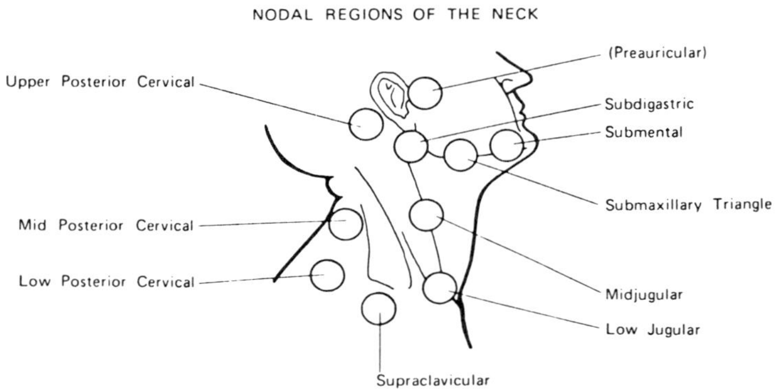

Figure 4.1. Nodal regions of the neck (from Fletcher).

PRETREATENT MANAGEMENT

Severe functional impairment of both temporary and chronic nature can be produced when head and neck tumors are irradiated. Most problems arise as a consequence of irradiating the salivary glands or mucous membranes. Diligent management must be undertaken before, during and following radiation.

Dental Prophylaxis

Dental prophylaxis is needed in patients receiving significant amounts of radiation to the salivary glands or mandible. Prophylaxis should include:

1. A dentist or oral surgeon should evaluate and restore carious and broken teeth. Extractions of non-restorable teeth should be performed with antibiotic (penicillin) coverage. At least 10 days post extraction healing prior to the initiation of radiation should be allowed. Full mouth extraction of restorable teeth is detrimental and must be avoided, since it increases oral trauma, delays initiation of irradiation and increases risk of osteonecrosis.

2. Dental hygiene instructions must be emphasized in order to maintain the teeth in the best possible state before, during and after treatment. A regimen of brushing 2-4 times daily with a soft brush, followed by oral lavage with a salt and bicarbonate solution (1 liter water + 5 cc sodium chloride + 5 cc sodium bicarbonate) and fluoride rinses (5 cc of 3% sodium fluoride).

3. A custom-made tray and fluoride gel should be provided for use 5 minutes after each brushing.

Nutritional Support

Nutritional support is important in all patients with head and neck cancers. Guidelines are:

1. Patient must avoid alcohol and cigarettes.

2. Calorie supplements and blenderized diets should be explained to the patient in order to maintain adequate nutrition.

3. Expect a weight loss of approximately 2 lbs weekly during radiation.

4. Hot and acidic fluids are to be avoided during radiation.

TREATMENT OF THE PRIMARY

EARLY LESIONS (T1, T2)

Radiation and surgery each can produce comparable cure rates for early head and neck cancers. Important factors to determine which modality to use may depend on:

1. Functional and cosmetic results: For example, an early laryngeal lesion treated with radiation results in a better preserved voice in a greater percentage of patients than with most surgical procedures.

2. General medical condition: Can the patient undergo surgical resection? Operative mortality overall may be low but may be greater in selected debilitated patients. Can the patient complete an extended course of radiation? The acute radiation reactions encountered are exacerbated by continued cigarette and alcohol abuse. Poor nutritional status may be further compromised by side effects of irradiation.

3. Salvage: Although initial local control may be equal with radiation or surgery, salvage is not. Early lesions initially irradiated can be surgically salvaged to a greater extent than those lesions initally resected can be salvaged with radiation. This may sometimes lend initial management with radiation therapy an advantage in overall local control.

4. Site of the primary: The primary disease may be relatively surgically inaccessible (e.g. nasopharynx) or accessible (e.g. tongue).

5. Treatment time: Surgery can usually be accomplished with a hospital stay of less than

two weeks. Radiation may require 6-8 weeks, although much or all of it may be administered as an outpatient.

6. Patient preference: The patient may prefer a particular treatment modality for other than the above reasons. It is important to recognize these reasons and give the patient as full an understanding of the treatment options as possible.

ADVANCED LESIONS (T3, T4)

A combined modality approach of radiation and surgery is often necessary to cure advanced cancers. The two modalities are complementary. Surgical treatment addresses gross disease adequately but may fail to encompass microscopic disease. Radiation can eradicate microscopic disease but may fail as the volume of gross disease increases.

Preoperative radiation is recommended if surgical resection is not possible. Advantages of preoperative radiation include:

1. Unresectable lesions may convert to resectable.
2. The extent of normal tissue resected may be diminished.
3. Distant metastases may be decreased.
4. Preoperative blood supply is better than postoperative, making the area more radiosensitive.

Postoperative radiation is given when the lesion is resectable, but the likelihood of microscopic residual disease is significant. The entire operative field may be at risk for recurrence due to possible surgical implantation. Advantages of postoperative radiation include:

1. A higher dose of radiation (6000 rad) can be given.
2. Surgical resection and healing take place more readily in non-irradiated tissue.
3. Additional pathologic information is available to better define tumor extent.
4. Tumor bulk is reduced.

Extent of surgery: When combined with radiation, the surgical procedure should be designed to remove gross disease only. More extensive procedures increase morbidity markedly.

For very advanced local disease, palliation may be the only reasonable approach. Unless the patient is in excellent medical condition, the significant morbidity and occasional mortality of aggressive combined therapies can outweight the poor chances for cure (often less than 5%).

TREATMENT OF THE NECK

The rich lymphatic supply of the head and neck region results in frequent spread of the primary malignancy into the neck. The risk of nodal involvement is dependent on the location, extent, and degree of differentiation of the primary tumor. The extent of neck disease correlates directly with the incidence of distant metastases and inversely with survival (less than 10% of patients presenting with an N0 neck develop distant metastases but nearly 40% develop distant metastases with an N3 neck). Death due to failure to control disease in the neck without concomitant failure at the primary site is unusual. Treatment of the neck in addition to providing improved local disease control may have some effect on survival, although this has not been shown conclusively.

The N0 Neck

The risk of developing neck node metastaes in a neck which is initially clinically N0 may be 30% or more Elective irradiation of clinically negative necks to 4500-5000 rad prevents the subsequent appearance of nodal disease in over 90% of patients irradiated. The whole neck is at risk for subclinical nodal disease when the primary disease is located in the nasopharynx, oropharynx or hypopharynx. For primary lesions which are small or lateralized in the oral cavity, glottic larynx or sinuses, treatment may be delivered to small volumes which may include only first echelon nodes at risk. Prophylactic treatment of the N0 neck with radiation offers control equal to or better than a radical neck dissection without significant disfigurement.

The Clinically Positive Neck

Radiation alone can control over 90% of neck nodes under 2 cm if treated to 6000 rad. As tumor bulk increases, the dose of radiation required for control increases and overall control diminishes. Approximately 7000 rad controls about 80% of 3 cm nodes. Occasionally, 3-4 cm nodes will disappear during the course of irradiation and surgery is not required. In particular, with primary tumors of the nasopharynx or tonsillar fossa a complete response to radiation often occurs even with advanced nodal disease.

In general, larger nodes (greater than 3 cm) should be managed with combined radiation and surgery if greater than 50% control is to be expected. Neck dissection for disease persisting in the neck after 5000-6000 rad should be carried out soon (within 4-6 weeks) after completion of radiation, since delay can result in fibrosis and make salvage surgery difficult.

Alternatively, a radical neck dissection may be carried out as the initial management of a clinically positive neck. A radical neck dissection is an extensive surgical procedure which sacrifices the sternocleidomastoid muscle, eleventh nerve, internal jugular vein and neck nodes. If multiple nodes are involved microscopically or if disease extends through the node, then postoperative radiation can significantly reduce local recurrence rates (from over 50% to less than 10%).

Cervical Nodal Metastases from an Unknown Primary Tumor

Metastases to lymph nodes of the neck is not an uncommon presentation encounted in clinical practice. Over 70% of patients with metastastic cancer in the neck have a primary tumor somewhere in the head and neck. Common occult sites of primary disease include the nasopharynx, tonsil and base of tongue.

Evaluation of patients presenting with neck metastases should include a thorough search for the primary lesion: a general physical exam with careful examination of the head and neck, a chest x-ray and other appropriate radiologic studies. If the inital exam fails to determine the site of the primary, the patient should undergo a direct head and neck exam under anesthesia with biopsies obtained from any abnormal mucosal surfaces. Random biopsies from the nasopharynx and occasionally from the base of the tongue, tonsil or pyriform sinus may reveal occult disease. An incisional, excisional or needle biopsy of the neck node, depending on the size, location and surgeon's preference, may be obtained to make the diagnosis. If a neck dissection is contemplated as a possible subsequent means of neck management then one should do either a needle biopsy or a biopsy with an incision that can be easily encompassed later in the neck dissection so as not to "seed" the neck with tumor.

The management of neck metastasis from an unknown primary is controversial. Knowlege of the patterns of lymph nodal drainage from head and neck sites is useful. Several management guidelines are offered:

1. Radiation therapy to the nasopharynx, base of tongue and neck has the potential of eradicating the occult primary as well as neck disease. In surgically treated patients, 20 to 30% subsequently manifest primary disease in one of these regions compared to less than 10% postirradiation.
2. Radiation therapy decreases the risk of contralateral neck metastases from 17% to essentially zero.
3. Supraclavicular metastases, particularly when adenocarcinoma, usually arise from sites below the clavicle and are associated with a poor prognosis (5-year survival 0-20%). Local irradiation to prevent progressive invasion can be given.
4. Patients with nodes in the posterior cervical triangle or with a positive EB virus titre have a high likelihood of an occult nasopharyngeal primary. They are best treated with radiation.
5. Patients with a single submaxillary or submental node are likely to have an oral cavity primary. Here, surgery with radiation salvage may be a reasonable alternative to initial extensive radiation.

In general, radiation therapy either alone (for small nodes) or in combination with surgery (for large nodes) offers a potential curative advantage over surgery alone in the management of neck nodes from an unknown primary. A five-year survival of about 50% can be obtained. The major disadvantage of extensive radiation (to potential primary sites as well as the neck) is that significant xerostomia may be induced. Individualized treatment weighing risks and benefits and using the guidelines presented above is suggested.

SPECIFIC SITES:TREATMENT AND RESULTS

An overview of management of primary lesions of specific sites is presented. One must remember that the neck must also be treated and such treatment may affect the type of therapy chosen for management of the primary disease also.

ORAL CAVITY

Lip, anterior two-thirds of tongue, floor of mouth, buccal mucosa, gingiva, retromolar trigone and hard palate.

Lip: Carcinomas of the lip usually arise on the mucosa or the vermillion border of the lower lip. They can be treated curatively with surgery or radiation in over 90% of patients. For small lesions (less than 1.5 cm), surgical resection may be preferred since it is as effective as radiation from a curative and cometic standpoint and does not require an extended treatment time. For moderately advanced lesions or lesions involving the commissure, radiation produces better cosmetic and functional results. Lymph node metastases, present in 10% of patients, occur in the submental and submaxillary regions.

Anterior two-thirds of tongue, floor of mouth: Early lesions (less than 1 cm) can frequently be successfully treated with either surgery or interstitial implant. Other T1 and T2 lesions may be managed radiotherapeutically with interstitial implant and external beam radiation. Local control with irradiation is greater than 75% for T1 and T2 lesions, and the majority of failures can be salvaged surgically. Initial surgical treatment is as successful as radiation in local control but cosmesis and function are usually worse and failures are less likely to be salvaged by radiation. Surgery is indicated when there is mandibular fixation, recurrence after radiotherapy, or for verrucous carcinomas or carcinomas arising from syphilitic glossitis. Lymph node metastases are frequently seen in the submandibular and upper and mid cervical nodes and must be included in treatment plans. Planned combined modality treatment is preferred for most advanced (T3 or T4) tumors though T3 oral tongue lesions may be treated successfully with radiation alone.

Buccal mucosa: Surgery or irradiation are curative for most early lesions. Radiation is preferred when there is involvement of the commissure or when a large skin graft might be required. External radiation with electrons can be used to spare contralateral normal tissue. Surgery is preferred when there is bone invasion. Lymph node metastases to the submandibular and subdigastric nodes occur in about 25% of patients (depending on primary size).

Gingiva, retromolar trigone, hard palate: Most lesions of these regions require surgical resection due to bony invasion. Radiation therapy can be used for early lesions without bony invasion with surgery for salvage, with local control of 80%.

OROPHARYNX

Base of tongue, tonsillar region, soft palate.

Base of tongue: Local control with radiotherapy alone is achieved in 60-80% of T1 to T3 tumors. Surgical salvage is rarely attempted due to morbidity and functional loss involved with a glossectomy and a laryngectomy after high dose radiation. Treatment of lymphatics is essential since even small lateralized lesions frequently have metastasized to ipsilateral and contralateral lymph nodes.

Tonsil: Radiation is the mainstay for all lesions of the tonsillar region. Local control for T1 and T2 lesions is 70-90% and salvage surgery is successful in about two-thirds of patients, so the ultimate local control is 90-96%. Larger T3 and T4 lesions are controlled 25-50% of the time with radiation. Surgical salvage in these larger lesions is more radical and is rarely attempted due to associated morbidity. Morbidity from radiation alone is predominantly xerostomia, although with early lesions (T1) treatment techniques can be used to spare the contralateral salivary gland since contralateral lymph node involvement is then infrequent.

Soft palate: The multifocal nature of cancers at this site usually preclude surgery. Radiation is successful in treatment of most lesions (T1 to T4) with 80-100% control rates.

HYPOPHARYNX

Pyriform sinus, pharyngeal walls, postcricoid area.

Pyriform sinus lesions comprise the great majority of hypopharyngeal lesions. Most hypopharyngeal cancers are advanced at presentation. Lesions of the apex or postcricoid area often have only indirect clinical findings, including pooling of secretions in the pyriform sinus region, arytenoid edema, and loss of laryngeal click. Radiation or partial laryngopharyngectomy can control 85-90% of T1 lesions. T2 and early T3 lesions are frequently treated with radiation, since operative mortality approaches 15% for total laryngopharyngectomy. Local control for advanced lesions (T3 and T4) treated with surgery and postoperative radiation is fair at about 40%, but five year survival is very poor, only about 15%, due to death from distant metastases, intercurrent disease, second primaries, and treatment complications.

NASOPHARYNX

Cancers of the nasopharynx are often not diagnosed until relatively advanced in part due to the difficulty in examining the area. Commonly, there is extensive local spread at presentation into the base of the skull, sphenoid sinus, retropharyngeal space, eustachian tube, nasal or paranasal sinus, or oropharynx. There is neck nodal involvement in 80-90% of patients on presentation with 50% bilateral nodes. Work-up must include CT scan to evaluate unsuspected disease extension. The incidence of subclinical nodal metastases is very high. Thus, the bilateral neck regions, including the posterior cervical chain, are always irradiated.

Overall survival with radiation is 60%. Early lesions without adenopathy can be cured in 80%. Advanced (T4) lesions with base of skull invasion have less than 25% five year survival with local control achieved in one-half of patients treated.

LARYNX

Supraglottis, glottis, subglottis (rare tumor).

Supraglottic larynx: Epiglottis, aryepiglottic folds, false cords, arytenoids.

Early lesions (T1, T2 and early T3) may be treated with either radiation or supraglottic laryngectomy with voice preservation and cure in 80%. Advanced lesions (T3 and T4) require surgery with preoperative or postoperative radiation. (An improvement in local control was seen with postoperative compared to preoperative radiation in RTOG study 73-03.) Survival at 3 years is about 50% and is dependent on neck node status.

Glottic larynx: T1 and T2 lesions of the true cords are best treated with radiation, since cure rates are good (80-90%) and voice preservation is better than with hemilaryngectomy or partial laryngectomy. With advanced lesions causing cord fixation (T3) or with lesions with extralaryngeal extension or cartilage invasion (T4), laryngectomy is usually used with postop radiation given for positive margins, subglottic extension, positive neck nodes, cartilage invasion or prior tracheostomy. Cure rates with this technique are in the 60-70% range. Alternatively, T3 lesions and selected T4 lesions can be treated initially with radiation to a dose of 4000 to 5000 rad. If fixation then persists, radiation is abandoned and surgery is undertaken. If the tumor regresses and there is a return of mobility, the treatment is continued to a full dose of 6800 to 7000 rad and the patient is closely followed and treated with salvage surgery if necessary. Using this approach about 50% of such T3 and T4 lesions can be cured with radiation alone. Of the patients that fail radiation, nearly 50% can be salvaged by laryngectomy. Therefore, this approach to advanced glottic cancer may be as effective as an initial surgical approach, yet offer the possibility of voice preservation in about 50% of the patients treated.

NASAL CAVITY, PARANASAL SINUSES

Lesions in these regions are usually advanced, bone involvement is frequent, and combined surgery and radiation are frequently needed. A line drawn between the inner canthus and the angle of the mandible divides the maxillary sinus into a <u>suprastructure</u> and an <u>infrastructure</u>. Early tumors of the infrastructure can be controlled in over one-half of patients. For larger tumors with invasion of the muscle and tumors of the maxillary suprastructure, cure rates are about 30%. Palliative irradiation may be useful to reduce pain, bleeding and proptosis.

SALIVARY GLANDS

Surgery is used in treating most major salivary gland malignancies. Postoperative radiation is indicated for high-grade lesions, close or positive surgical margins, recurrent tumors, tumors of the deep lobe, and regional nodal disease. Cure rates depend on histology. One-third of undifferentiated tumors are cured compared to three-fourths of low-grade mucoepidermoid tumors.

EAR

Cancers of the ear can be divided into three categories based on anatomic location and response to radiation.

<u>Pinna</u>: Fractionated orthovoltage radiation can produce excellent control and cosmesis of skin cancers of the pinna even if cartilage is invaded.

<u>Auditory canal (outer two-thirds)</u>: Tumors of this region are rare. They are usually squamous cell carcinomas. CAT scans aid in the defining of extent of disease. Radiotherapy can control early tumors with good cosmesis and little morbidity.

<u>Auditory canal (inner one-third), middle ear, mastoid air cells</u>: These tumors are usually advanced squamous cell carcinomas at presentation. Attempts at surgery with postoperatie irradiation have produced five year survivals of 33-45%. If there is extension beyond the temporal bone, there is virtually no chance

for control. Death is usually attributable to invasion of the brain.

MORBIDITY

The following is a list of reactions that may occur during or after head and neck irradiation. Keep in mind that the reactions are seen only if the normal tissue in question is being irradiated. For example, treatment of laryngeal tumors involve none of the reactions below except laryngeal edema, since essentially only the larynx is being treated.

Acute Reactions

1. Mucositis: A mucosal radioepithelitis appears about 12-17 days after the initiation of radiation. This exudative reaction can progress from patchy to confluent mucositis. (Interestingly, the region of the tumor sometimes undergoes an early "tumoritis", or pseudoexudative reaction, just several days after radiation initiation, thus aiding in identification of tumor versus normal mucosa). If the mucositis is non-confluent, it can be managed with continued saline and bicarbonate lavage and analgesics such as acetaminophin. Temporary ulceration may occasionally occur after 3000 rad. Glyceride and viscous xylocaine are useful in relieving oral discomfort. A confluent mucositis will require a break in radiation treatments. Mucosal healing occurs rapidly (several days) after radiation cessation. About 2-3 weeks are necessary for complete healing after a full course of radiation therapy.

2. Parotitis: Occasionally, patients will complain of a painful, swollen parotid gland occurring approximately 8-12 hours after the first radiation treatment. This is related to radiation-induced inflammatory changes in the parotid and usually resolves within a few hours. Aspirin may be used for persistent symptoms.

Acute and Chronic Reactions

1. Xerostomia: When most of the salivary glands, particularly the parotids, are irradiated, the saliva diminishes and thickens. Such changes can be noted within the first week of treatment. Two thousand rad can cause clinically noticable temporary salivary impairment and over 4000 rad will probably result in permanently decreased salivation. Glyceride, baking soda and carbonated drinks may improve acute problems of thickened, tenacious saliva. Salivary substitutes are available for chronic xerostomia. Loss of adequate saliva to lubricate food, dilute and buffer acids and cleanse the oral cavity can lead to multiple problems including dental caries.

2. Loss of taste: During the acute mucosal reaction, some patients will complain that foods have lost their flavor. Much of this is due to xerostomia and mucositis and eventually will be recovered. However, taste buds can also be damaged by radiation. Sour and bitter tastes are suppressed more than sweet and salty. The degree of taste loss correlates best with xerostomia.

3. Otitis externa, otitis media: Inflammatory changes in the ear canal and middle ear are commonly seen at doses above 4000 rad. They occur during treatment or soon thereafter and are manifested by pain, infection and decreased hearing. Cortisporin may be useful in otitis externa. Decongestants are very useful for middle ear problems but occasionally myringotomy may be necessary to relieve discomfort.

Chronic Reactions

1. Osteonecrosis of the mandible: Radiation affects bone by injuring the small vasculature of the Haversian system and the periosteum as well as direct osteocytic damage. This diminishes the bone's ability to withstand

trauma and avoid infection. The overall incidence of radio-osteonecrosis is less than 2% but is dose dependent and rises to nearly 10% for doses over 7000 rad. Important risk factors include poor nutrition, poor oral hygiene, trauma, continued smoking, and alcohol consumption. Additionally, when the primary tumor is large or is located in or close to bone, as with floor of mouth tumors, the incidence rises to nearly 25%. If attempts to conserve teeth fail, post-irradiation dental extractions must be done extremely judiciously, choosing patients without risk factors, since extractions may initiate osteonecrosis. A conservative approach of meticulous hygiene is necessary to avoid an infection, which may expand the area of necrosis and cause pain. A gentle removal of loose bony spicules can be attempted. Topical or systemic antibiotics may be indicated if infection is present. If the patient does not respond to conservative treatment within a reasonable period or has increasing pain, a trial of hyperbaric oxygen may result in significant pain relief and improvement. If hyperbaric oxygen is not available, then a surgical resection of irradiated mandible may be indicated.

2. Soft tissue necrosis: This rare complication occurs most often secondary to an ill-fitting prosthesis or a very high local dose of irradiation, as may be delivered with an interstitial implant. Since the mucosa and gingiva continue to change up to several months following irradiation, it is best to avoid making a new prosthesis for at least 3 months following completion of radiation. Any ill-fitting prosthesis is a continued source of irritation and should not be used. Conservative management, including oral hygiene, antibiotics and occasionally hyperbaric oxygen, is usually adequate for healing, if the necrosis is not due to recurrent tumor.

3. Radiation dental caries: Pretreatment dental management and prophylaxis, along with fluoride usage, minimizes this problem. The mature tooth is radioresistant, though the peridontal membrane and pulp vasculature can be injured and result in loosening and loss of the tooth.

4. Trismus: Fibrosis around the masticatory muscles can result in trismus. It can be due to radiation alone, but is more frequently seen when postoperative radiation is given. Stretching exercises may be effective in improving this problem.

5. Fibrosis: Subcutaneous fibrosis may occur in any irradiated area, but typically is most severe in the neck, particularly when combined with a neck dissection. Some submental edema (turkey waddle) develops and usually subsides after several months. Exercise prevents contractures.

6. Endocrine dysfunction: The hypothalamus, pituitary or thyroid may be included in the radiation portal in the treatment of some head and neck tumors. Endocrine abnormalities can be seen clinically when the dose to these glands exceeds 4000 rad and over 3/4 of the gland has been irradiated.

7. Laryngeal edema: Edema of the arytenoids may occur after a course of radiation to the larynx and may be managed conservatively by voice rest, antibiotics for ulceration, and perhaps steroids. If edema persists for more than 3 months following completion of radiation, the majority of these patients will be found to have recurrent or persistent tumor. Since the tumor usually recurs submucosally, a biopsy, even if deep, may be negative for tumor and additionally may worsen the edema. Usually a laryngectomy will be required for management.

8. Myelitis, cataracts, second malignancy: These are covered elsewhere. Please see appropriate chapters.

CHEMODECTOMAS

Carotid body, glomus, jugulare tumors.

These slow-growing tumors of paraganglia are considered benign since they rarely metastasize but frequently they can produce symptoms referable to local growth and invasion. A familial pattern has been described.

Carotid body: Unless discovered early when they can be safely surgically excised, treatment should not be attempted.

Glomus jugulare: Glomus tumors often exhibit aggressive local behavior and usually recur post-surgically. Symptoms of local progression and invasion, including tinnitus, bleeding, decreased hearing, can be stablized or improved with relatively low does of radiation (4000 rad).

MIDLINE GRANULOMA

This is a locally progressive destructive disease of the upper air passages. Pathologically one sees necrosis, small vessel vasculitis, granulomas, and chronic inflammation. It may be the same disease as lymphmatoid granulomatosis. It must be differentiated from malignant lymphoma as well as Wegener's granulomatosis. Unlike Wegener's granulomatosis, it rarely involves the lungs or kidneys and rarely is associated with disseminated small vasculitis. If untreated, death ensues from meningitis, hemorrhage or malnutrition. External beam radiation to the upper respiratory passages may produce excellent long-term control in 80% of patients with localized disease. Multifocal disease responds poorly even with the addition of steroids plus or minus cytoxan.

THYROID

A subtotal thyroidectomy is the procedure of choice for patients with papillary follicular thyroid carcinoma. Patients over age 40 should have an I-131 tracer study two to three days postoperatively to determine if residual thyroid disease remains. External beam radiotherapy may be used to treat patients with residual carcinoma that does not take up I-131. If I-131 is taken up by residual thyroid tissue, an ablative dose of I-131 is given and the patient is placed on thyroid hormone replacement. This procedure is repeated every four to six months until all thyroid uptake is ablated or a total of 500 mCi of I-131 is given. Initial I-131 treatment which delivers 30,000 rad to the thyroid, is recommended for successful therapy. Follow-up I-131 scans are then indicated every six to twelve months for three negative scans. Patients under age 40 are placed on thyroid hormone suppression doses of T3 or T4. Most endocrinologists choose to use T4 over T3 since it is less expensive, has less hyperthyroid effects and can be used once a day (T3 given is TID). Patients with anaplastic thyroid carcinoma are treated palliatively with radiotherapy alone or in combination with Adriamycin.

REFERENCES

1. Fletcher G, Jesse R: The place of irradition in the management of the primary lesion in head and neck cancers. Cancer 39:862-872, 1977.
2. Fletcher GH: Elective irradiation fo subclinical disease in cancers of the head and neck. Cancer 29:1450-1454, 1972.
3. Wang C: Radiation therapy for head and neck cancers. Cancer 36:748-751, 1975.
4. Strong E: Pre-operadiation and radical neck dissection. Surg Clinics of North America, vol 49 no 2, 1969.
5. Maxon H, Thomas S, Hertzberg V: Relation between effective radiation dose and outcome of radioiodine therapy for thyroid cancer. N Eng J Med 309:937-941, 1983.

Chapter 5

Central Nervous System Tumors

TUMORS OF THE BRAIN

OVERVIEW

Primary tumors of the brain pose a challenge to the oncology team because of their anatomic location and the delicate nature of nervous tissue. The neurosurgeon often finds these tumors inaccessible for biopsy or only incompletely resectable. Because the brain is confined by the bony calvarium, a histologically benign tumor can behave malignantly. It has been estimated that the lethal tumor burden in the brain is 100 grams, while the lethal burden for systemic cancer is 1 kilogram. Radiation, therefore, plays an indispensible role in the management of many CNS lesions. Only primary brain tumors will be considered below by histologic diagnosis. Cerebral metastases are discussed in Chapter 16, dealing with palliative radiotherapy.

PATHOLOGY

Primary intracranial neoplasms may arise from:

1. Glial or astrocytic elements (astrocytomas, oligodendrogliomas and ependymomas)
2. Primitive neuronal elements (medulloblastomas)
3. Pia arachnoid (meningiomas)
4. Schwann cells of cranial nerves (neurilemomas)
5. Blood vessels (hemangioblastomas)
6. Remnants of Rathke's pouch (craniopharyngiomas)
7. Neurendocrine tissue (pituitary adenomas)
8. Intracranial connective tissue (primary brain sarcomas)
9. Intracranial lymphatic tissue (primary brain lymphomas)
10. Remnants of the notochord (chordoma) and embryonal cell rest (pinealomas, dysgerminomas)

Gliomas, accounting for 50% of all primary brain tumors, have classically been characterized by the Kernohan grading system (Grades I-IV). Recently, the classification of gliomas has been modified with three subgroups: Astrocytoma, astrocytoma with anaplastic foci (AAF) and glioblastoma multiforme (GBM). The distinction between AAF and GBM is made chiefly on the basis of the microscopic presence of necrosis in GBM. Prognostically, the new classification is more reliable. Table 5.1 lists the frequency of primary brain tumors in adulthood and childhood.

Table 5.1
Approximate Frequency of Primary Brain Tumors

Type	Adulthood	Childhood
Glioblastoma Multiforme	25%	10%
Other Astrocytomas	25%	20-30%
Oligodendroglioma	2-3%	2%
Ependymoma	2-6%	12-16%
Medulloblastoma	1%	20%
Meningioma	15%	2-6%
Pituitary Adenoma	10-15%	1-2%
Optic Glioma	0-1%	5%
Craniopharyngioma	1-2%	12%
Brain Stem Glioma	1-2%	10-15%
Miscellaneous	5-10%	5-10%

CLINICAL FEATURES

The symptomatology of intracranial neoplasms is often determined by the tumor location. These symptoms are usually insidious in onset and their progression is determined by the growth kinetics of the mass lesion. Headaches commonly occur and are worse in the mornings. If headaches are localized, there is some correlation with tumor location, e.g., suboccipital headaches suggest posterior fossa tumors while headaches involving the vertex are seen with pituitary tumors. Investigation of unexplained seizure activity in adults uncovers an intracranial neoplasm in a third of such patients. Increased intracranial pressure caused by mass effect of a brain tumor with a surrounding area of edema or from obstruction to the outflow of CSF from the ventricular system manifests itself as headache, nausea, vomiting and alterations in mental status. Papilledema is present in as few as 25% of these patients. Unilateral deafness is a hallmark for the acoustic neuroma. Impotence can be an initial complaint in patients with prolactinomas. Other syndromes include galactorrhea-amenorrhea, Cushing's syndrome, gigantism and acromegaly. Endocrine dysfunction manifests itself as hyper or hyposecretion of hormones as a presenting sign of pituitary tumors. Infratentorial tumors often present with signs and symptoms related to obstructive hydrocephalus, cerebellar dysfunction and cranial nerve involvement.

Because of their strategic location, small pituitary tumors may cause visual complications due to compression of the optic chiasm.

STAGING

A TNM classification has been proposed but is not in widespread clinical use.

WORK-UP

When a diagnosis of primary brain tumor is suspected on the basis of history, a thorough neurologic examination is essential in an effort to localize the lesion. Diagnostic testing may include:

1. Computerized tomographic scanning: The availability and noninvasive nature of CT scanning has established this technique as the mainstay of diagnosis, largely supplanting echoencephalography and pneumoencephalography. CT scanning will be used increasingly for radiation treatment planning purposes to minimize irradiation of normal structures and still maintain adequate margins about the tumor.
2. Routine skull films: Since the advent of CT, these are often neglected but can provide valuable information, particularly regarding calcification of tumors such as craniopharyngiomas, meningiomas and oliogodendrogliomas.

3. Cerebral arteriography: This remains valuable especially when surgical intervention is planned and also to rule out vascular lesions which may present as intracranial masses.
4. Radionuclide brain scan: This is still more available than CT scanning and is positive in approximately 85% of patients with primary brain tumors.
5. NMR scanning: The role of this new diagnostic modality remains to be defined.

TREATMENT AND RESULTS

LOW GRADE GLIOMAS

For incompletely resected lesions, postoperative radiotherapy has been shown to prolong disease-free survival in patients with low-grade gliomas. Postoperative radiotherapy involves irradiating various volumes of brain tissue to 4000-5000 rad with a field reduction to the tumor volume for another 500-1500 rad. Some authors treat limited volumes throughout the course of radiotherapy. These policies can be expected to result in a five-year survival of 60% for incompletely excised grade I astrocytomas and 25% for incompletely excised grade II gliomas. For grade I cerebellar astrocytomas, which have undergone complete excision, survival is quite excellent with an 85% ten-year survival rate without adjuvant radiotherapy.

ASTROCYTOMAS WITH ANAPLASTIC FOCI (AAF)/ GLIOBLASTOMA MULTIFORME (GBM)

Resection directly correlates with survival time. Postoperative radiotherapy must be regarded as palliative even when combined with radiation sensitizers and/or chemotherapy. Prolongation of life is measured in months rather than years. Age and initial performance status are strong prognostic variables. The standard therapy is to deliver 6000 rad to the whole brain over a 6-7 week period. Again, the treatment of smaller volumes is being investigated, using CT treatment planning. Aggressive multimodal therapy in patients with AAF yields a median survival of 27 months and a five-year surival of 10-20%. For patients with GBM, this regimen will yield a median survival of 8 months, with essentially no five-year survivors.

Research efforts to improve survival in this devastating illness include high LET irradiation, hypoxic cell radiosensitizers, combination chemotherapy administered systemically or via selective intra-arterial infusion, interstitial brachytherapy and interstitial hyperthermia.

MEDULLOBLASTOMA

Surgery alone is rarely, if ever, curative due to the proclivity of this cerebellar tumor to seed the CSF pathways. The goals of surgery are _diagnosis_, _decompressive_ and _tumor debulking_. CSF-system shunts should be avoided as they are thought to contribute to metastases. Nevertheless, systemic metastases have been recognized without shunting procedures. When decompression cannot be accomplished surgically, _ventriculostomy_ is to be preferred.

Postoperative radiotherapy involves _total craniospinal axis irradiation_ after maximal surgical tumor removal. Since medulloblastomas chiefly occur in a pediatric population, special technical considerations are involved. For very young children, general anesthesia may be required. Encompassing the requisite volume of tissue is very demanding both on the technical staff whose responsibility it is to irradiate the cranium and spine without unacceptable high dose areas where fields overlap and on the patient who must receive radiotherapy to 40-50% of active bone marrow. The technique of avoiding field overlap involves a series of junctions which are shifted periodically throughout the treatment. The doses commonly employed are 5000-5500 rad to the posterior fossa, 4000-5000 rad to the whole brain and 3500-4500 rad to the spine. _Myelography should be performed on all patients with abnormal CSF cytologies_. The dosages to the spine are generally determined by the presence or absence of tumor cells in the CSF (best determined by sampling fluid from the lumbar sac rather than ventricular fluid) and the presence or absence of gross tumor deposits seen at myelography. The myelogram is abnormal in approximately 35% of patients with abnormal cytologies. Sites of gross tumor nodularity are boosted to higher doses.

Collin's rule has been applied to medulloblastoma. This states that patients who are disease-free for a period equal to their age at diagnosis plus 9 months are cured of their tumor. Five-year survival rates range from 40-60%.

OLIGODENDROGLIOMA

This gliomatous tumor is characterized by a slow growth with a pattern of late recurrence. Often they occur mixed with elements of higher grade astrocytomas. Management is identical to that of low grade gliomas. The addition of postoperative radiation therapy approximately doubles the five-year survival from surgery alone to about 80%. Because of late relapse, the 10-year survival is only 30%.

EPENDYMOMA

Pathologic grading of these intracranial tumors is essential to treatment planning. Complete resection is unusual and postoperative radiotherapy is indicated. Lower grade ependymomas are treated like other low-grade gliomas with local radiotherapy to 5000 rad. High grade ependymoblastomas are managed like medulloblatomas. Again, CSF cytology and myelography play a role in treatment planning. The 5-year survival figures with a combined surgery and postoperative radiotherapy regimen range from 45-75%.

MENINGIOMAS

Meningiomas are usually histologiclly benign and are, therefore, cured when surgical resection is complete. The indications for postoperative therapy are:

1. Total excision is not possible.
2. The tumor is histologically malignant.
3. The tumor is already recurrent.

Doses of 5000-6000 rad delivered using local fields can delay or prevent recurrences in these situations. For incompletely resected meningiomas, Wara and associates have reported a 30% recurrence rate with postoperative irradiation versus 74% without it.

PITUITARY ADENOMA

For patients with pituitary tumors, surgery may be employed to confirm the clinical diagnosis and as primary therapy. The choice of the surgical approach is often dictated by tumor size. A transfrontal approach is preferred when there is significant suprasellar or lateral tumor extension, although it is accompanied by higher morbidity and mortality. When possible, transsphenoidal hypophysectomy leads to remission in most patients. When there is rapid progression of visual symptoms (decreasing visual acuity or increasing scotomata), increased intracranial pressure or cranial nerve deficits, decompressive surgery is required. If excision has been incomplete, postoperative radiotherapy can control tumor growth.

Radiotherapy alone can be used to treat pituitary tumors. A dose of 4500 rad is delivered to the pituitary tumor and is sufficient to destroy tumor with a very low incidence of hypopituitarism. There may be a 2-4 year delay in the decline of hormone levels caused by hyperfunctioning pituitary adenomas. This delay makes transsphenoidal hypophysectomy the treatment of choice for hyperfunctioning intrasellar tumors. Proton beam irradiation has also been used in treating these tumors because of its more favorable dose distribution (See Chapter 20). In general, the mortality from pituitary adenomas is low with five-year survivals reported in the 80-95% range. Recent reports hold promise for the use of dopamine agonists such as bromocriptine and pergolide for the therapy of patients with prolactin-secreting macroadenomas and acromegalics. Suppression of both serum prolactin concentration and serum growth hormone levels have been demonstrated with concomitant tumor shrinkage demonstrated by serial CT scanning. This approach remains investigational.

CRANIOPHARYNGIOMA

These pediatric tumors arising from the remnants of Rathke's pouch are either solid tumors of columnar cells or cystic tumors lined with squamous epithelium. Complete surgical excision is often difficult owing to the tumor size and involvement of neighboring vital structures. Postoperative radiotherapy is designed to deliver 5500-6000 rad over a 7 week period to the pituitary region using an arc technique or a three field cross-fire plan. This policy will result in a 5-year disease-free survival of approximately 85%.

PINEAL REGION TUMORS

Tumors located in the pineal region are rare and are usually inaccessible to biopsy because of their deep location. The differential diagnosis would include gliomas, dysgerminomas and metastases. Radiotherapy can be used to help differentiate these histologic types. Following 2500-3000 rad whole brain irradiation over a two and a half week to three week period, a CT brain scan is repeated. If there has been a dramatic response, this is presumptive evidence that the pineal tumor is the more radioresponsive dysgerminoma. Dysgerminomas are prone to CSF seeding and there is rationale for proceeding with craniospinal irradiation. If a glioma is suspected, 5000-6000 rad is delivered to the pineal area. Five-year survivals for dysgerminomas approximate 75%.

HEMANGIOBLASTOMA, NEURILEMOMAS, PRIMARY BRAIN SARCOMA

Hemangioblastomas are vascular tumors, which are characteristically slow growing, cystic and primarily involving the cerebellum and are to be distinguished from vascular malformations. Surgery is the treatment of choice but if they recur irradiation can be given. These tumors are often seen in association with the Lindau-von Hippel syndrome. Intracranial neurilemomas are tumors formed from Schwann cells of cranial nerves. Most commonly, the 8th nerve is involved an the tumors are located in the cerebellopontine angle (CPA). These tumors are best approached surgically. They may occur as single lesions but are also found to be multiple in association with neurofibromatosis. Malignant Schwannomas are locally invasive and have the capacity to metastasize. The application of radiotherapy to these malignant tumors has not been widespread. Primary brain sarcomas are seen in children and young adults and are treated with surgery and postoperative local field irradiation. Metastases outside the CNS can occur.

OPTIC PATHWAY GLIOMA

These tumors are usually well-differentiated astrocytomas, which extend along the optic nerve intracranially causing enlargement of the optic foramen and involvement of the optic chiasm and hypothalamus. Management consists of transcranial inspection and biopsy (if vision will not be compromised), followed by postoperative radiotherapy with the goal of preserving sight. A dose of 5500 rad in over six weeks is delivered to local fields. The five-year survival is approximately 80% with 75% of these patients having maintained or improved visual status.

BRAIN STEM GLIOMA

This common pediatric brain tumor has primarily been managed by a radiotherapeutic approach. Presently the diagnosis can be made on the basis of history, clinical findings and CT scanning. Craniotomy yields tissue suitable for diagnosis less than 60% of the time. In the case of cystic or exophytic tumors, surgery offers short-term benefit and is also occasionally required for shunt placement in patients with hydrocephalus. Radiotherapeutic management consists of treatment of the primary site (as defined by CT scan) wiht generous margins, delivering 5000-5500 rad in 5-6 weeks. When planning treatment portals, the possibility of extension to the hypothalamus and upper cervical spinal cord must be kept in mind. Most series report 5-year survival of approximately 30%.

THALAMIC AND MID-BRAIN TUMORS

These tumors frequently occur in childhood with an equal sex ratio. The symptomatology is similar to brain stem tumors with increased intracranial pressure causing headache, nausea and vomiting. Cranial nerve deficits are seen in the majority of patients. Biopsy is again considered to carry risk of substantial morbidity. The primary management remains radiotherapeutic and surgery should be limited to shunting procedures. Of 14 patients treated with radiation therapy (5000-5500 rad in 5-6 weeks) at the Harvard Joint Center for Radiation Therapy, 6 patients are free of disease greater than 5 years after treatment. Five-year survival in the literature ranges from 37% to 72%.

PRIMARY BRAIN LYMPHOMA

Primary large cell "histiocytic" lymphoma of the central nervous system often referred to as reticulum cell sarcoma of brain or microglioma, is a rare tumor commonly associated with renal transplantation, Wiskott-Aldrich syndrome, ataxia-telangiectasia and the acquired immunodeficiency syndrome (AIDS). A recent report suggests induction of this lymphoma by Epstein-Barr virus. The goal of neurosurgical management is to establish the tissue diagnosis and to resect the tumor if this can be accomplished without resulting neurologic deficits. Corticosteroids will often yield a dramatic clinical improvement accompanied by objective responses as documented by serial CT scans. The roles of radiotherapy and chemotherapy are not well defined since the tumor is so rare and there have been few long-term survivors to date. When radiotherapy is employed, whole brain irradiation should be given since marginal recurrences have been reported when smaller volumes are treated. Since this disease entity was first described in 1929, only a handful of patients have survived for more than 5 years free of disease.

MORBIDITY

Acute

In general, whole brain irradiation in the clinical dose range is well tolerated but symptoms such as headache, nausea and somnolence occasionally occur. These radiation-induced acute symptoms can be ameliorated by the use of corticosteroids and are probably related to cerebral edema and changes in vascular permeability. Epilation and radiodermatitis are also seen during radiotherapy and are dose-related phenomenon. Alopecia will be permanent in most patients receiving doses greater than 5000 rad. A skin reaction tends to be worse near the pinnae, the forehead and occiput, which are irradiated tangentially by lateral portals.

Early Delayed Radiation Injury

The appearance of neurologic signs and symptoms during the first two to three months following completion of radiotherapy for intracranial tumors has been referred to as "early delayed injury" and has been attributed to transient radiation demyelination.

Late

Brain necrosis may appear months to years following high dose irradiation of the brain (5000-7000 rad). The exact etiology of chronic radiation injury to the CNS remains controversial, with some investigators favoring primary parenchymal injury and others attributing late effects to blood vessel damage. Kramer and Sheline and associates have studied this clinical problem extensively by reviewing all cases of bona fide brain necrosis following radiation therapy that have been reported in the literature. On the basis of these studies, Sheline estimates that a dose of 5200 rad in 26 fractions over 5 weeks will lead to cerebral necrosis in less than 1% of patients. It is often difficult to differentiate late brain necrosis from tumor recurrence, although CT scanning and cerebral arteriography may be helpful. Leukoencephalopathy has been reported in leukemic children treated with cranial irradiation and both intrathecal and systemic methotrexate. It is rarely seen with radiotherapy alone.

Using sophisticated psychometric testing, subtle intellectual impairment has been demonstrated in children receiving cranial irradiation as part of their neoplastic management. The developing central nervous system is undoubtedly more sensitive to ionizing radiation than the adult brain. Recently, similar degrees of impaired cortical function have been described in two groups of children with brain tumors receiving radiotherapy. The first group were patients with medulloblastoma receiving craniospinal irradiation while the second group consisted of patients with cerebellar astrocytomas who received only posterior fossa irradiation. It is implied that the cerebral dysfunction may be related to increased intracranial pressure rather than the effects of radiotherapy.

Pituitary irradiation can lead to optic nerve and chiasmal damage in 2-13% of patients depending on the daily fractionation. Hypopituitarism and the empty sella syndrome have also been reported.

Craniospinal irradiation for medulloblastoma and ependymoblastoma will have delayed effects, some of which depend upon the patient's age at the time of therapy. These include growth disturbances in the irradiated bones and the development of second tumors (e.g. thyroid).

TUMORS OF THE SPINAL CANAL

OVERVIEW

Spinal canal tumors account for 20% of central nervous system tumors with a frequency of 4000 new cases per year. These tumors may be (1) intradural and intramedullary, (2) intradural but extramedullary and (3) extradural and extramedullary. Because all these tumors directly involve or are adjacent to critical neural tissue, complete excision may not be possible. Postoperative radiotherapy would, therefore, be indicated.

PATHOLOGY & CLINICAL FEATURES

Ependymomas and astrocytomas account for most intramedullary spinal cord tumors. Intraspinal glioblastoma multiforme are rare and account for only 1.5% of all spinal cord tumors. Schwannomas and meningiomas account for 50% and are found in intradural, extramedullary locations. Most extradural spinal canal tumors are of metastatic origin and will be discussed in Chapter 16 dealing with radiotherapeutic emergencies. Chordomas arising from notochordal tissue remnants may occur extradurally along the craniospinal axis, with 50% located in the sacrococcygeal area, 15% in the vertebral area and 35% in the basisphenoid area. Adequate surgical removal of chordomas is rarely possible. Of all intraspinal tumors, 6-8% are vascular and include hemangioblastomas and hemangioendotheliomas. Epidermoid and dermoid cysts are rare entities.

Signs and symptoms of spinal canal tumors will depend upon location. Pain of gradual onset and progressive in nature is an early symptom and can be localized to a particular level of the spine. This may be followed by radicular pain. Other symptoms include paresthesias, limb weakness and unsteadiness of gait. Disturbances of bowel and bladder function occur late in the course. Primary intramedullary astrocytomas and ependymomas tend to have a prolonged clinical course with occasional spontaneous improvement.

WORK-UP

Neurologic exam may show signs of a single nerve root involvement with hyporeflexia and weakness in a segmental distribution. Hypesthesia may be found in the appropriate dermatome distribution but major sensory loss is a late finding. Spinal cord involvement yields hyperreflexia, Babinski signs, spastic weakness, bilateral sensory findings below the level of the lesion and sphincter dysfunction. Involvement of the cauda equina will produce lower extremity hyporeflexia, bilateral flaccid weakness, multiple dermatomal sensory deficits and urinary retention with overflow incontinence. Meningiomas and Schwannomas, which are lateralized, often present as the Brown-Sequard syndrome caused by transverse hemisection of the spinal cord, thus causing ipsilateral upper motor neuron paralysis and ipsilateral loss of vibratory and position sense but contralateral loss of pain and temperature sensation below the level of the lesion.

When a diagnosis of spinal cord tumor is entertained, a lumbar myelogram is indicated. If a block to he flow of contrast material is identified, cissternal puncture is necessary to define the upper extent of the block. High-resolution CT scan is also valuable.

TREATMENT AND RESULTS

Intramedullary astrocytomas and ependymomas: The role of surgery is that of establishing a tissue diagnosis and providing decompression. Total excision is rarely possible without incurring major neurologic deficits. Postoperative radiotherapy to a dose of 5000 rad is generally recommended. For low-grade ependymomas, the prognosis is usually somewhat better than their intracranial counterparts with five-year survivals in the order of 83%. Spinal cord astrocytomas treated in a similar fashion will have 5-year survivals greater than 50%.

Meningioma and Schwannomas are benign tumors with total surgical excision remaining the treatment of choice.

Chordomas: Patients with these tumors are generally referred to the radiotherapist following biopsy alone or incomplete resection. Postoperative radiotherapy has been shown to be effective in providing palliative tumor growth restraint with subsequent relief of symptoms. Few patients are cured, with five-year disease free survival ranging from 5-10%. Some authors recommend high doses doses of radiotherapy (> 7000 rad) but this approach carries risk of significant morbidity and adequate palliation has been claimed with more moderate doses ranging from 4000 to 5500 rad by conventional fractionation. For clivus tumors, the use of proton beam irradiation is being explored at the Massachusetts General Hospital but results are preliminary. Multiple fractions per day are also being tried with encouraging results.

MORBIDITY

Acute

Transient radiation myelopathy is an occasional mild, temporary post-radiation phenomenon. This is characterized by paresthesias and Lhermitte's sign. This sign is elicited by neck flexion, which produces electric shock-like sensations in the arms and legs. This will occur 2-4 months following irradiation administration for diseases such as Hodgkin's disease, esophageal carcinoma, bronchogenic carcinoma and head and neck tumors. The syndrome may be self-limiting with spontaneous recovery being the rule; however, it may be the first sign of late cord damage. It is postulated that transient radiation-induced myelopathy is related to depression of myelin synthesis with latent period related to myelin turnover.

The acute effects of craniospinal irradiation are related to the volume of bone marrow encompassed in the fields with leukopenia and the thrombocytopenia commonly occurring. Pharyngeal irrritation and nausea are also seen.

Late

Delayed or irreversible myelopathy is a dread complication with a latent period ranging from 6 months to several years. At times it is related to technical errors when matching portals over the spinal cord. It may be seen with uncoventional dose fractionation. Clinically, it manifests itself as ascending paresthesias, spastic motor paralysis and disturbances of bowel or bladder function. When incomplete transverse myelitis is present, the findings of the Brown-Sequard syndrome are present. The lesion is due to necrosis of white matter with small blood vessel pathology. A spinal cord dose of 5000 rad given by conventional fractionation of 900-1000 rad per week is generally regarded as safe. The diagnosis of radiation myelopathy is one of exclusion since recurrence of a spinal cord tumor or the developement of an extradural metastases can present an identical picture. Myelography is therefore indicated. A recent case report documented an intramedullary tumor metastasis simulating radiation myelitis with a normal myelogram, but this is a rare phenomenon.

REFERENCES

1. Chang CH, Horton MD, Schoenfeld D et al: Comparison of postoperative radiotherapy and combined postoperative radiotherapy and chemotherapy in the multidisciplinary management of malignant gliomas. Cancer 52:997-1007, 1983.
2. Sheline GE: Radiation therapy of tumors of the central nervous system in childhood. Cancer 35:957-964, 1975.
3. Garret PG and Simpson WJK: Ependymomas: results of radiation treatment. I J Rad Onc Bio Phys 9:1121-1124, 1983.
4. Cummings BJ, Hodson D, Bush RS: Chordoma: the results of megavoltage radiation therapy. I J Rad Onc Bio Phys 9:633-642.
5. Danoff BF, Kramer S, Thompson N: The radiotherapeutic management of optic nerve gliomas in children. I J Rad Onc Bio Phys 6:45-50, 1979.
6. Littman P and Wang CC: Reticulum cell sarcoma of the brain. Arch Neurol 35:1975.
7. Lambert, PM: Radiation myelopathy of the thoracic spinal cord in long term survivors treated with radical radiotherapy using conventional fractionation. Cancer 41:1751-1760, 1978.

Chapter 6

Eye and Orbital Tumors

OVERVIEW

Diseases of the eye and orbital contents treated by radiotherapy are relatively uncommon. They include benign diseases such as pterygium, orbital pseudotumor, Graves' exophthalmos and others. Malignant diseases in adults include orbital and choroidal metastases, lacrimal gland tumors, carcinoma of the bulbar conjunctiva, orbital lymphomas and melanomas. Pediatric malignancies include retinoblastomas, optic nerve gliomas, and orbital rhabdomyosarcomas. Orbital irradiation may result in a variety of normal eye and orbital tissue responses. Those responses may occur when irradiating the eye or orbital diseases listed above or non-orbital primary tumors, such as nasal cavity and paranasal sinus tumors.

BENIGN DISEASES

Pterygium: These fibrovascular proliferations of the bulbar conjunctiva recur after surgical excision in 20-40% of patients. Postoperative beta irradiation initiated within 2-48 hours of excision can reduce recurrence to 5-10%. A second course of excision and postoperative radiation is successful in salvaging 80% of the few patients that fail the initial course of treatment. The beta irradiation is given by means of a strontium-90 applicator placed in contact with the eye. Several radiation schemes exist, some utilizing a single treatment but most employing several fractions over a 1 to 3 week period starting within 2 days of excision. Doses of 2000 to 3000 rad to the conjunctiva and pterygium bed are typically given. Due to the limited penetration of the beta ray the dose to the lens is low (<90 rad) and clinically important cataract formation is uncommon.

Orbital pseudotumor: This nonspecific chronic inflammatory disease can mimic Graves' exophthalmopathy in its clinical presentation (particularly when bilateral) with proptosis, periorbital swelling and impairment of eye movement. The diagnosis can be (but is not always) established by biopsy with diffuse lymphocytic infiltration seen histologically. CT scan is essential since CT findings are distinctly different from Graves' ophthalmopathy. With orbital pseudotumor, muscle enlargement is often asymmetric and located posteriorly at their insertions. Frequently the retro-orbital fat and posterior globe structures are obliterated. In contrast, Graves' ophthalmopathy usually produces symmetric anterior muscle enlargemnt with preservation of posterior globe structures. Steroid therapy can be very beneficial but long-term use is frought with side effects. Recurrence after surgical excision is frequent. External beam radiotherapy (2000 rad in 10 days) can bring about a rapid resolution of orbital pseudotumor with excellent tolerance and low recurrence risk and appears to be a preferrable alternative to surgery or steroid treatments.

Graves ophthalmopathy: Most cases of exophthalmos due to hyperthyroidism do not require therapy. Steroids may be used in patients with severe symptoms. Ophthalmopathy not responding to steroid treatment may respond to radiotherapy. More than half the patients have a good to excellent response with radiation of 2000 rad in 2 weeks. Response to radiation appears to be better in those who develop symptoms rapidly compared to those with longstanding or slowly-developing symptoms.

Other benign diseases for which radiotherapy is sometimes used include the treatment of:

1. Juvenile hemangiomas when persistent or progressive and symptomatic.
2. Histiocytoses and eosinophilic granuloma with exophthalmos.
3. Angiomatosis retinae (von Hippel-Lindau) with extensive or progressive retinal involvement.

4. Herpes zoster with involvement of the ophthalmic branch of the fifth nerve (radiation must be given soon after the appearance of the first papules to be effective).

ADULT MALIGNANT DISEASES

Adult Choroidal Metastases: Metastasis to the choroid represents the most common adult orbital tumor, estimated to occur in 5% of patients with known metastatic cancer. Breast cancer is the most frequent primary site (comprising over 80% of cases), followed by lung. The disease is unilateral in two-thirds of patients. Radiation can improve vision in two-thirds of patients and deterioration of vision can be prevented in most others. Duration of response of patients with choroidal metastases is nearly the same as their median survival, which is about one year. Doses of 3000 rad in 2 weeks and 4000 rads in 3 weeks to the choroid have frequently been used. Techniques may be employed to avoid treatment of the lens in patients with a relatively long estimated life expectancy (e.g. 12 months).

Lacrimal gland: Like salivary gland tumors, primary treatment is surgical. Unfortunately, surgical treatment results in a low cure rate. Postoperative radiotherapy indications are the same as for salivary gland tumors (See Chapter 4). Advanced unresectable lesions may benefit from radiation therapy alone.

Conjunctival cancers: These rare lesions are usually superficial squamous cell carcinomas that can be adequately treated with external beam orthovoltage radiation therapy alone. Surgery is reserved for advanced lesions with ocular infiltration.

Lymphoma: Orbital non-Hodgkin's lymphomas may be the only manifestation of lymphoma or they may be part of a generalized lymphoma. Staging work-up should be the same as for non-Hodgkin's lymphomas presenting at other sites (See Chapter 8). External beam radiotherapy results in excellent local control. Since prospects for long-term survival are good, radiotherapy techniques must be chosen to minimize long-term morbidity. Five-year actuarial survival rates of 70-80% have been reported.

Melanoma: Melanomas may occur intraocularly, originating in the choroid, or may occur on the conjunctiva. Choroidal melanomas can be seen on ophthalmoscopic exam as a pigmented mass extending from the choroid into the vitreous cavity. Pathologically, the epitheloid cell melanoma fares poorly compared with the spindle cell variant.

Conjunctival melanomas can be removed surgically. Residual disease responds to either external beam or strontium-90 radiation.

Choroidal malignant melanomas are presently treated according to size: For _small tumors_ (less than 10 mm in diameter, less than 2 mm elevation) the choice of management is affected by factors such as degree of visual impairment, rapidity and extent of progression, age of the patient, and vision in the opposite eye. Management options vary from observation to local therapy (radiotherapy, cryotherapy, xenon, photo-coagulation, argon laser therapy, etc.) to systemic therapy (chemotherapy or immunotherapy) to enucleation. Treatment of _medium size tumors_ (10-15 mm in diameter, 2-5 mm elevation) is controversial but observation only is not recommended as it sometimes is for small tumors. _Larger tumors_ (greater than 15 mm. in diameter, 5 mm elevation) are treated with enucleation. Some authors have noted an increase in mortality due to metastases following enucleation and attribute this to dissemination at the time of surgery.

Although melanomas are relatively radioresistant, intraocular melanomas are not radioincurable. Radiation can be delivered by cobalt-60 (Stallard plaque) temporarily sutured to the eye with over two-thirds of patients with small to medium tumors having a complete response. Proton beam irradition has also been used and is successful in the treatment of small tumors.

PEDIATRIC MALIGNANT DISEASES

Retinoblastoma: This intraocular neoplasm in children is discovered at an average age of 18 months. Two-thirds are unilateral and one-third are bilateral at presentation or within 18 months. Retinoblastoma can occur as a spontaneous mutation or, in about 10% of patients, as an autosomal dominant. Familial retinoblastoma is transmitted in an autosomal dominant fashion with 80% to 90% penetrance. The majority of patients with a family history of retinoblastoma have bilateral disease.

The Reese classification (See Table 6.1) groups the disease by prognosis. It is useful for treatment planning and gives a general idea of the natural history of the disease.

Table 6.1
Reese Classification of Retinoblatoma

Group I: Very favorable
1. Solitary tumor, less than 4 disc diameter in size, at or behind equator.
2. Multiple tumors, none over 4 disc diameter in size, all at or behind equator.

Group II: Favorable
1. Solitary tumor, 4 to 10 disc diameter in size at or behind equator.
2. Multiple tumors, 4 to 10 disc diameter in size behind equator.

Group III: Doubtful
1. Any lesion anterior to the equator.
2. Solitary tumors larger than 10 disc diameter behind equator.

Group IV: Unfavorable
1. Multiple tumors, some larger than 10 disc diameter.
2. Any lesion extending anteriorly to ora serrata.

Group V: Very unfavorable
1. Massive tumors involving over half of retina.
2. Vitreous seeding.

The majority of patients have multifocal disease in one or both retinas. Enucleation is used in patients with advanced disease with little or no useful vision, as is usually the case in spontaneous unilateral tumors. When disease is found early, as with patients with a family history of previous retinoblastoma, external beam radiation can be highly successful with 70-90% tumor control with useful vision.

Orbital rhabdomyosarcoma: Children with orbital rhabdomyosarcoma require radiation as the mainstay of treatment. Local control can be achieved in the majority of patients if proper treatment techniques are utilized. (See Chapter 15)

Optic nerve glioma: Radiation therapy has been used to succesfully control these lesions when surgery is inadvisble (e.g. vision present but extension of disease to chiasm precludes surgery). Recently, results of treatment with chemotherapy suggest that it also may be effective in controlling growth of these tumors.

MORBIDITY OF ORBITAL RADIATION

The post-treatment management of patients who have received orbital irradiation can be difficult. An ophthalmologist who is familiar with and interested in radiation complications should evaluate patients before treatment.

Cataracts: The lens is sensitive to radiation. Cataracts due to radiation are seen as opacities near the posterior pole. Their posterior subcapsular position is identical to non-radiation induced cataracts. Treatment is the same as for non-radiation induced cataracts, i.e. removal as necessary. The latent period is more than a year and at low doses (250-650 rad) is about 8 years. A single dose as low as 200 rad can produce a cataract. Several factors are important in radiation cataractogenesis:

1. Dose-time-fractionation. As with most normal tissues, a given dose produces less of an effect if given in more fractions, spread over a longer period of time. When treatment is

spread over several weeks, several hundred rad may be necessary to produce a cataract. Virtually all patients will develop a cataract with total doses of more than 1000 rad. Yet clinically important cataracts with significant visual loss occur in only 10% of adults treated with high dose radiation to the eye.

2. Age. Sensitivity of the lens decreases with age. The elderly not only have a lower incidence for a given dose of cataract formation than children but also the latent period for development is longer, often several years.
3. Type of radiation. Neutrons are more effective in producing cataracts than gamma or x-irradiation. (An RBE of more than 20 is probable).
4. Administration of chemotherapy. When 5-FU is given concomitantly with radiation to high doses, over half the patients may develop clinically important cataracts.

Conjunctivitis: Inflammation of the conjunctiva is commonly seen with doses of 3000-4000 rad or more but may occur even at doses of 1000 rad. Onset is usually within 2 to 3 weeks following completion of radiation. Conservative treatment with steroid based ophthalmic solutions will ease discomfort.

Keratitis: This corneal problem may occur together with conjunctivitis. Tiny punctate ulcers on the anterior surface of the cornea can be seen when stained with fluorescein. Treatment is conservative as with conjunctivitis.

Ulceration: Areas of keratitis may coalesce to form corneal ulcers in 10-15% of patients with high dose radiation (6000 rad or greater). They appear between 4 months and 1 year following irradiation. Steroid should not be used for radiation induced corneal ulcers. Referral to an ophthalmologist is necessary for proper management.

Sicca: Dry eye results when the lacrimal gland is irradiated to over 4000 rad. This is a very serious problem which could result in loss of the eye. Therefore, care must be taken to avoid this by shielding the lacrimal gland from the radiation. Artificial tears should be used if diminished lacrimation is noted.

Epilation: Doses of over 2000 rad can produce permanent loss of the eyelashes. With sparing of superficial tissue seen with megavoltage radiation, the eyelashes may remain intact even after 5000 to 6000 rad are given to deeper structures.

Eyelid Atrophy: High doses of radiation may cause tarsal atrophy and thinning but usually does not result in functional impairment.

Epiphora: Excessive tearing due to stenosis or obstruction of the nasolacrimal duct is rarely caused by radiation alone. It may be seen following radiation if there has been prior disruption of drainage by tumor or surgery.

Retinal damage: Radiation-induced changes in the small retinal vessels can produce retinopathy and retinal atrophy with gradual visual loss. The clinical picture is similar to that of diabetic retinopathy. Retinal changes resulting in decreased visual acuity may be seen with fractionated doses as low as 1000 rad. However, clinically significant retinal atrophy does not usually develop with doses of under 5000 rad. Clinical expression of retinal injury does not occur until approximately 18 months following irradiation. Visual acuity is normal until that time, then over a several month period progressively deteriorates. Elderly and diabetic patients may be at increased risk for radiation-induced retinopathy. Thrombosis of the central retinal artery results in sudden blindness and is seldom seen with doses under 6000 rad.

Optic nerve damage: Two major types of post-radiation optic nerve injury are described: (1) Ischemia injury due to small vessel changes resulting in distal nerve injury and (2) retrobulbar optic neuropathy due to proximal nerve injury (without disc edema or hemorrhage). Optic nerve atrophy may occur at higher doses (over 6000 rad), and take somewhat longer to develop (2-5 years) than retinal atrophy.

Glaucoma: Neovascularization of the anterior surface of the iris due to radiation may produce secondary angle closure glaucoma. Rarely, radiation may change the permeability of uveal vessels and produce an iridocyclitis resulting in glaucoma. Conservative treatment of glaucoma may be attempted but enucleation may eventually be needed.

REFERENCES

1. Donaldson S et al: Supervoltage orbital therapy for Graves' opthalmopathy. J Clin Endocrin 37:276-285, 1973.
2. Bahrassa F and Datta R.: Postoperative beta radiation treatment of pterygium. I J Rad Onc Bio Phys 9:679-684, 1983.
3. Chan RC and Shukousky LJ: Effects of irradiation on the eye. Radiology 91: 116-120, 1968.
4. Enzman D et al: Computed tomography in orbital pseudotumor and computed tomography in Graves' opthalmopathy. Radiology 120:597-601 and 615-620, 1976.
5. Halnan KE: Tumors of the eye treated with radiation therapy. Clin Radiology 13:19-29, 1962.
6. Parsons JT et al: The effects of irradiation on the eye and optic nerve. I J Rad Onc Biol Phys 9:609-622, 1983.
7. Reese AB: Tumors of the eye. N.Y. 1963. Harper and Row, Publishers Inc.
8. Chu FC et al: Radiation therapy of choroid metastasis from breast cancer. I J Rad Onc Bio Phys 2:273-279, 1977.

Chapter 7

Breast Cancer

OVERVIEW

There are multiple approaches to the management of breast cancer at present. The role of radiation therapy is manifold: primary, preoperative, postoperative and palliative. Treatment techniqiues will continue to evolve, particularly as we better define the effectiveness of adjuvant chemotherapy in preventing both distant metastases and local-regional recurrence.

PATHOLOGY

Certain pathologic features influence the natural history and prognosis in breast cancer patients; these include (1) size of the primary lesion, (2) regional nodal status, (3) microscopic features (such as histologic subtype, grade, blood vessel or lymphatic invasion) and (4) estrogen receptor (ER) protein status.

The size of the primary lesion correlates directly with the risk of axillary lymph node metastasis and local recurrence. For example, a 1 cm primary is associated with a 20% risk of axillary metastasis and less than 5% local recurrence rate compared to a 45% axillary metastases risk and 20% local recurrence rate for a 5 cm primary.

The status of regional lymph nodes is the most important single factor in determining prognosis. The 5 year disease-free survival decreases from nearly 80% in patients without axillary metastases to 48% in patients with 1-3 nodes involved and 33% in patients with 4 or more nodes involved. Adjuvant chemotherapy has improved disease-free survival in node positive patients by about 15%.

The histologic subtype, grade, lymphatic infiltration and blood vessel invasion may be of prognostic significance. The majority of breast cancers are infiltrating ductal adenocarcinomas (80%). Others include medullary (7%), invasive lobular (5%), mucinous (2.4%) and tubular (1%). Medullary carcinoma (even with positive nodes) and tubular carcinoma (which has a low incidence of nodal involvement) may have a better prognosis than other invasive breast cancers. Microinvasive carcinomas have a 1-3% incidence of nodal involvement. Ductal carcinoma in situ (1%), and lobular carcinoma in situ (1%), rarely if ever, metastasize to nodes or beyond. Paget's disease of the nipple (2%) is frequently associated with in situ or infiltrating ductal carcinoma elsewhere in the breast. The diagnosis of inflammatory breast cancer is a clinicopathologic one. It includes the clinical findings of skin erythema, warmth and induration and the pathologic findings of tumor cells in dermal lymphatics. Inflammatory breast cancer is associated with a very poor prognosis.

The estrogen receptor status has a general prognostic value and is also therapeutically important primarily in the palliative management of disseminated or advanced disease. Relapse-free survival is superior in women with ER positive tumors compared to women with ER negative tumors. Knowledge of estrogen receptor status is important in determining palliative response to hormonal manipulation. There is about a 60% chance that a response will be obtained in a patient with an ER positive cancer compared to only 8% chance in ER negative cancers. The ER status does not appear to predict the response to chemotherapy.

CLINICAL FEATURES

Breast cancer is the most common malignancy in women over age 40. The risk of developing breast cancer is increased in patients with a family history of breast cancer and nulliparous patients. Female to male ratio is 100:1. Cancer in the opposite breast will eventually manifest clinically in about 6% of patients.

Typically, the patient presents with a lump in the breast which in early stages is small and mobile. Advanced cancer may cause ulceration, fixation to skin, muscle or ribs, pain, retraction of the skin or nipple, erythema and axillary nodal masses. Rarely, symptoms referable to distant metastases (bone, pleural or pulmonary) will be the presenting complaint.

STAGING: (Clinical-Diagnostic Classification)

Note: Clinical assessment does not always correlate well with pathologic findings. For example 20-30% of clinically suspicious axillary nodes are pathologically negative and up to 40% of clinically negative axilla contain pathologically positive nodes. Therefore, treatment should be based on both clinical and pathologic assessment.

T-Primary Tumor

TIS-Carcinoma in situ
(Note: Paget's disease with a demonstrable tumor is classified according to the size of the tumor)

- T0: No demonstrable tumor.
- T1: Tumor 2 cm. or less in greatest dimension.
  - T1a: No fixation to underlying fascia and/or muscle.
  - T1b: Fixation to underlying fascia and/or muscle.
- T2: Tumor 2-5 cm. in greatest dimension.
  - T2a: No fixation to underlying fascia and/or muscle.
  - T2b: Fixation to underlying fascia and/or muscle.
- T3: Tumor > 5 cm. in greatest dimension.
  - T3a: No fixation to underlying fascia and/or muscle.
  - T3b: Fixation to underlying fascia and/or muscle.
- T4: Tumor of any size with direct extension to chest wall or skin.
  - T4a: Chest wall fixation.
  - T4b: Edema, infiltration, or ulceration of skin of breast (including peau d'orange), or satellite skin nodules confined to the same breast.
  - T4c: Both of the above.
  - T4d: Inflammatory carcinoma

<u>N-Regional Lymph Nodes</u>

N0: No palpable ipsilateral axillary nodes.

N1: Movable ipsilateral axillary nodes.

N1a: Nodes not considered to contain growth.

N1b: Nodes considered to contain growth.

N2: Ipsilateral axillary nodes fixed to one another or to other structures.

N3: Ipsilateral supraclavicular or infraclavicular nodes or edema of the arm.

<u>M-Distant Metastases</u>

M0: No evidence of distant metastases.

M1: Distant metastases present.

<u>Stage Groupings</u>

Stage I:	T1a, N0 or N1a M0
	T1b, N0 or N1a
Stage II:	T0, N1b, M0
	T1a, N1b, M0
	T1b, N1b, M0
Stage II:	T2a, N0 or N1a or N1b, M0
	T2b, N0 or N1a or N1b, M0
Stage III:	Any T3 with an N, M0
	Any T4 with any N, M0
	Any T with N2, M0
	Any T with N3, M0
Stage IV:	Any T, any N with M1

WORK-UP

Physical exam, bilateral mammogram or xeromammogram, biopsy (incisional or excisional depending on management approach-see below), chest x-ray, CBC, SMA-12 (special attention to liver chemistries, calcium, alkaline phosphatase) are required for the initial work-up.

A single mass, or a recently appearing mass, especially in older women should be evaluated by a biopsy even if the mammogram is negative. Aspiration in lieu of biopsy should be used only when the mammogram is negative for cancer, the mass completely disappears after aspiration and close follow-up can be obtained.

Though bone scans are still standard work-up for breast cancer, only about 2 to 3% of all patients will have detectable bone metastases at the time of diagnosis.

TREATMENT AND RESULTS

EARLY CANCER: Stage I (T1, N0) and Stage II (T1,2 and N1).

Surgery

The present standard operation in this country for early tumors is the modified radical mastectomy with axillary lymph node dissection. This procedure is now preferred over radical mastectomy for most resectable breast cancers since it offers the same cure rate, but with the modified radical mastectomy the pectoralis major muscle is preserved, and there is less extensive skin and axillary dissection. Therefore, there is less major long term morbidity - less lymphedema of the arm and better cosmesis. Additionally, reconstruction of the breast is easier following modified radical mastectomy.

Adjuvant Chemotherapy

Patients with pathologically involved axillary nodes receive adjuvant chemotherapy to prolong disease-free survival and improve overall survival by controlling subclinical distant metastases and also to prevent local-regional recurrences. The use of the adjuvant combination chemotherapy, CMF, (cytoxan, methotrexate, 5-FU) or similar drug combinations in node positive patients improves relapse-free survival over untreated controls by about 15% overall. This is apparent by 3 years following initial treatment and (at last analysis) is still maintained at over 7 years.

This survival benefit has been demonstrated in pre-menopausal patients and may also occur in post-menopausal patients who receive an adequate drug dose (85% or greater of prescribed dose). Six cycles of CMF may be as good as 12 cycles. Though single agent adjuvant chemotherapy may offer a survival advantage to node positive premenopausal patients it is inferior to combination chemotherapy and, therefore, has no role in the present adjuvant managment of breast cancer. The adjuvant use of hormonal agents in addition to chemotherapy is being studied. The use of chemotherapy in node negative patients, particular in those patients who are also ER negative, is also under investigation.

Postoperative Radiotherapy

Adjuvant postoperative radiotherapy following mastectomy significantly reduces chest wall and regional nodal recurrences, particularly in patients at a high risk for local-regional recurrence such as those with extranodal or multiple axillary nodal involvement, large primary lesions (over 3 cm.) positive surgical margins, and skin or muscle involvement. However, there is little evidence to suggest that preventing the manifestation of local-regional disease with adjuvant radiotherapy significantly impacts on survival. Since there is no increase in cure rate the use of postoperative radiation is no longer routine. Postoperative radiation may be useful when given alone in selected patients with moderate to high risk of local-regional recurrence, or when given in addition to chemotherapy (again to prevent local-regional recurrence only). The effectiveness of adjuvant chemotherapy alone in preventing local-regional recurrence, particularly in patients with a high risk of local-regional failure, has not been clearly demonstrated.

Primary Radiotherapy

An effective alternative to mastectomy in many patients with early cancers of the breast combines excisional biopsy, axillary dissection, and primary radiotherapy. The resulting local-regional control and survival at five and ten years is equal to more radical surgical procedures.

Most patients with early breast cancer who desire to preserve their breasts are candidates for primary radiotherapy. However, patients with multiple primary lesions where excision of each lesion would result in unacceptable cosmesis should not be offered primary radiotherapy. Additionally, patients with larger T_2 lesions (4 to 5 cm) in small breasts would not be acceptable candidates for this technique.

1. Excisional Biopsy: Bilateral mammograms must be obtained prior to excisional biopsy to define location and limits of the tumor and rule out multiple primary lesions. It is important for the radiotherapist to see the patient before excisional biopsy so that he

may: (1) Determine whether the patient is an acceptable candidate for radiotherapy. (2) Note location and size of tumor for future treatment reference. (3) Discuss the treatment and results, including morbidity, with the patient.

Excisional biopsy should remove all gross disese with an approximate 1 cm. margin. If gross disease is not completely removed, the dose of radiation required to obtain local control may result in unacceptable cosmesis. Microscopically positive margins do not appear to effect local control, though most radiotherapists use a somewhat higher total dose when a microscopically positive margin is obtained. Metallic clips should be placed at the margins of the excised tumor to aid the radiotherapist in his treatment. Tissue should be sent for hormone receptor status.

2. Axillary Dissection: An evaluation of axillary nodes is necessary for prognostic information and to determine if there is a need for adjuvant chemotherapy particularly in the premenopausal patient. One may elect to spare selected post-menopausal patients from axillary dissection, e.g. those with clinicly negative axilla who might have difficulty tolerating chemotherapy. An axillary dissection which includes level I or levels I and II (to the medial border of the pectoralis minor muscle) gives sufficient information regarding the axillary nodal status. At least 6 and preferrably 10 or more nodes should be obtained in order to assess nodal status. Less than 1% of patients will have metastases to level III nodes in the absence of level I and II nodal involvement.

3. Radiotherapy: The delivery of adequate radiotherapy and use of good treatment techniques are required to produce both optimum local control and cosmesis. Radiation usually begins about 2 to 4 weeks following breast biopsy and axillary dissection. The patient by then has good arm mobility and can be easily placed in a treatment position.

External beam radiation of 4500-5000 rad in five weeks via tangential opposed fields is used to treat the breast. Beam modifiers such as wedges must be used to deliver a homogenous dose. Inclusion of regional nodes in the treatment field varies with tumor location and axillary nodal status.

The region of the excised primary receives an additional boost radiation dose of 1200-2200 rad with either electrons or via implant of iridium-192. Some institutions do not deliver this additional radiation if the margins of resection of the excised primary are microscopically negative. The choice of an electron boost or implant may be the result of technical factors. For example, a lesion excised from the inner quadrant close to the chest wall would probably be treated with electrons, since an implant there may be technically difficult or may deliver an excessive dose to the chest wall. If an implant is chosen, it may be done under general anesthesia at the time of axillary dissection or, more commonly, following external beam radiation. Frequently, it can be done on a cooperative patient under local anesthesia. The implant remains in place two to three days and generally does not require analgesics. Electron boosts can be done as an outpatient, are very well tolerated, and require one to two weeks of treatment.

4. Chemotherapy: Patients who have positive axillary nodes and are candidates for adjuvant chemotherapy may receive this before, during or after the radiotherapy. The acute effects of radiation, particularly on the skin, are exacerbated when concomitant chemotherapy is given. Therefore, some institutions omit one or more chemotherapeutic agents during radiation (e.g. Cytoxan and 5-FU is given instead of Cytoxan, Methotrexate, 5-FU and Prednisone). The sequencing of chemotherapy and radiation is presently being studied.

Primary Radiotherapy Results

As mentioned, the results of local-regional control and survival are the same with conservative surgery and primary radiotherapy as with more radical surgery. (See Table 7.1)

Table 7.1
Local Control and Survival with Primary External Radiation Therapy

		5-year	10-year
Local Control	T_1	92%-98%	90%-95%
	T_2	85%-90%	85%
Survival	Stage I	85%-90%	70%
	Stage II	70%	50%

Cosmetic results are influenced by the extent and location of the biopsy procedure as well as the radiation technique. Results are regarded as good to excellent in over 85% of patients. Less than 5% of patients develop significant breast fibrosis or permanent edema.

LOCALLY ADVANCED CANCERS: Stage III (T3, T4, or N2) and Stage IV (T4 or N3)

Patients with locally advanced breast cancer have a high likelihood for local-regional recurrence following mastectomy (40-60%) and a poor prognosis (5-year survival of 25-50%). The optimal sequencing of local and systemic treatment has yet to be determined. Radiotherapy may be used as follows:

Preoperatively: In patients with unresectable tumors, preoperative radiotherapy of 5000 rad in five to six weeks may allow surgical resection. If preirradiation chemotherapy is given to increase control and prolong survival, care must be taken to avoid excessive morbidity. Adriamycin and methotrexate may significantly increase skin reactions and combined treatment modalities may produce a greater degree of myelosuppression.

Postoperatively: Patients with advanced but resectable tumors need postsurgical treatment with radiotherapy to decrease local recurrence. Effective chemotherapy is needed additionally to attempt to improve survival as well as decrease local recurrence. The optimal sequencing of these modalities needs to be individualized.

Primary Radiotherapy: A reasonable level of local control (equal to that following mastectomy) can be obtained with excisional biopsy and radiotherapy (75%) even for advanced tumors (e.g. T3, N0). Adequate doses of radiation (over 6000 rad) must be delivered to achieve such control. If gross residual disease remains postexcision, an interstitial implant must be used to achieve similar control. Relapse-free survival is poor (20-30% at 5 years) due to the high likelihood of occult distant metastases. Addition of chemotherapy may improve five year relapse-free survival to over 50%, but this has not been firmly established.

STAGE IV BREAST CANCER (with distant metastases):

Palliation of advanced metastatic breast cancer can be achieved by hormonal manipulations. Factors associated with favorable response to hormonal manipulations include estrogen and progesterone receptor positive tumors, soft tissue rather than visceral metastases, a long (>2 year) disease-free interval (i.e. the interval between the treatment of the primary disease and the appearance of metastases), and prior response to hormonal management.

Breast: Radiotherapy may be used to provide local control and palliation of the primary breast disease in patients with distant metastases. Generally it is witheld if the patient is to receive systemic chemotherapy in order to evaluate response without surgery or radiation.

Brain: Cranial irradiation of 3000 rad in two weeks may produce improved or stable neurologic state, improved clinical status, and relief of headache. Overall median survival is about five months. The cause of death may be related to brain metastases despite cranial radiation in one-third to one-half of patients treated.

Bone: Palliative radiotherapy of painful bony metastases results in pain relief in over 80% of patients treated. Pathologically fractured bones should be surgically stabilized if possible. Radiotherapy is given postoperatively.

Other sites: See palliation chapter, (Chapter 17).

LOCAL REGIONAL RECURRENCE

Chest wall and nodal recurrences can be a serious problem since they may result in bleeding, ulceration and pain. Radiation therapy can result in complete response in 60-70% of patients, but overall local control is only 40-50% due to re-recurrence. Survival following local recurrence is poor with only a 20% five year survival and a median time to distant metastases of 12-15 months. Improved survival is seen in patients with a long disease-free interval between mastectomy and initial recurrence and in patients who have a complete response to treatment of the recurrence. Chemotherapy given after local-regional failure has not been shown to improve survival but should be considered.

MORBIDITY

Primary Radiotherapy

Acute and chronic morbidity from primary radiotherapy are minimal when careful surgical and radiotherapeutic approaches are applied. Chemotherapy may accentuate radiation reactions.

Acute: Post-surgically the patient may develop a hematoma, seroma or induration in the axilla or at the breast biopsy site. Cellulitis is rare but should be avoided since it can result in a frozen shoulder. During radiation the patient may experience some fatigue and temporary skin reactions which may vary from erythema to moist desquamation and rarely to skin ulceration (reversible).

Chronic: As previously mentioned, cosmesis is usually excellent with very limited induration of the breast if any when primary radiotherapy is utilized for early breast cancer. Primary radiotherapy for advanced breast cancer is associated with a greater incidence of breast fibrosis due to higher doses used. Chronic complications are rare. Chondritis, osteitis or rib fractures may be seen when high local doses are given as when an implant is placed close to bone or cartilage. Symptomatic pneumonitis occurs in less than 5% of patients treated and is related to treatment of the lung apex included in the supraclavicular/axillary field used in patients with positive nodes. Asymptomatic apical pulmonary fibrosis may also be seen if a supraclavicular/axillary field is used. Arm edema, brachial plexopathy and soft tissue necrosis are rarely seen with standard doses. When doses exceed 7000 rad, breast necrosis, nerve damage and soft tissue necrosis may occur in over 15% of patients.

Primary radiotherapy does not compromise adequate administration of adjuvant chemotherapy, that is, the percentage of patients receiving optimal chemotherapy (> 85% of prescribed dose) is no less following primary radiotherapy than following mastectomy.

Pre and Postoperative Radiotherapy

Again, morbidity from radiation prior to or following a mastectomy is dependent on the radiation technique as well as the surgical procedure performed. Mild to moderate late skin changes of telangiectasia, induration and change in pigmentation are frequently seen. The incidence of arm edema is increased over surgery alone if the axillary and supraclavicular regions are irradiated. As with primary radiotherapy, pneumonitis may occur and depends on the volume of lung irradiated.

Theorized Morbidity

Second malignancy induction: The incidence of carcinoma in the contralateral breast is the same whether the patient receives mastectomy, excisional biopsy and primary radiotherapy, or postoperative radiotherapy (about 6%). There have been no cases of radiation-induced sarcoma reported following primary breast irradiation despite its usage (in a modified form) since the early 1930's. Sarcomas, particularly lymphangiosarcomas, have been reported following postoperative chest wall radiation but have also been reported following radical mastectomy alone.

Depression of immune response: No study has shown that radiotherapy of breast cancer results in diminished survival due to radiotherapeutic depression of the immune response. More specifically, prospective serial studies have failed to demonstrate that minor temporary alterations in circulating lymphocyte subpopulations or in immune response have had any deleterious effects.

REFERENCES

1. Bonadonna G, Valagussa P: Chemotherapy of breast cancer: Current views and results. I J Rad Onc Bio Phys 9:279-297, 1983.
2. Chu FC, Lin F, Kim J et al: Locally recurrent carcinoma of the breast. Cancer 37:2677-2681, 1976.
3. DeLena M, Fucali R, et al: Combined modality approach in locally advanced breast cancer (T3b-T4). Proc Am Soc Clin Onc, 1976.
4. Hellman S, Harris JR, Levene MB: Radiation therapy of early carcinoma of the breast without mastectomy. Cancer 46:988-994, 1980.
5. Host H, Brennhoud I.: The effect of post-operative radiotherapy in breast cancer. I J Rad Onc Bio Phys 2:1061-1067, 1977.
6. Legha SS, Davis HL, Muggia FM: Hormonal approaches in breast cancer: new approaches and concepts. Ann Int Med 88:69-77, 1978.
7. Rose C, Botnick L, Weinstein M, Harris J, Koufman C, Silen W, Hellman S: Axillary sampling in the definitive treatment of breast cancer by radiotherapy and lumpectomy. I J Rad Onc Bio Phys 9:339-344, 1983.
8. Weichselbaum R, Marck A, Hellman S.: The role of postoperative irradiation in carcinoma of the breast. Cancer 37:2682-2690, 1976.

Chapter 8

Lymphomas and Hematologic Malignancies

HODGKIN'S DISEASE

OVERVIEW

Hodgkin's disease is now curable in the vast majority of patients due to advances in diagnosis, staging and treatment. Forty years ago the median survival of this disease, when untreated, was under one year. Since then, overall cure rates have improved from less than 20% to over 75%. Improved cure rates are largely the result of better diagnosis and staging, improved radiotherapy equipment (allowing the delivery of higher doses with less morbidity) and the development of effective combination chemotherapy. The treatment techniques which have evolved since then are sophisticated and require much attention to detail if failures and complications are to be minimized.

PATHOLOGY

Hodgkin's disease is probably a disease of T-lymphocyte origin. Its diagnosis depends upon identification of the Reed-Sternberg cell- a large cell with two or more nuclei, each containing a single prominent nucleolus. The Rye modification of the Lukes and Butler classification (1966) designates four histologies: lymphocyte predominance, nodular sclerosis, mixed cellularity, and lymphocyte depletion. The reproducibility of this classification among pathologists is about 70%. Nodular scerosis and mixed celluarity make up 70-80% of all cases.

CLINICAL FEATURES

There is a bimodal distribution in the incidence of Hodgkin's disease, with one peak at age 15-34 and the other at age 50 and above. In contrast to non-Hodgkin's lymphoma, Hodgkin's disease commonly is localized and involves contiguous axial nodes. Approximately 50% of patients have mediastinal involvement. Involvement of peripheral nodes (e.g. epitrochlear, popliteal), Waldeyer's ring and mesenteric nodes are rare. Liver and bone marrow involvement also are rare without B symptoms. If the liver is involved, the spleen is almost always involved.

The stage distribution is: I, 15%; II, 40%; III, 35% and IV, 10%. Less than 10% of stage I patients have B symptoms compared to over 80% with stage IV. Lymphocyte predominance and nodular sclerosis usually present with early disease, whereas lymphocyte depletion is usually more advanced.

STAGING

The Ann Arbor Classification (1970) relies on both clinical and pathologic data.

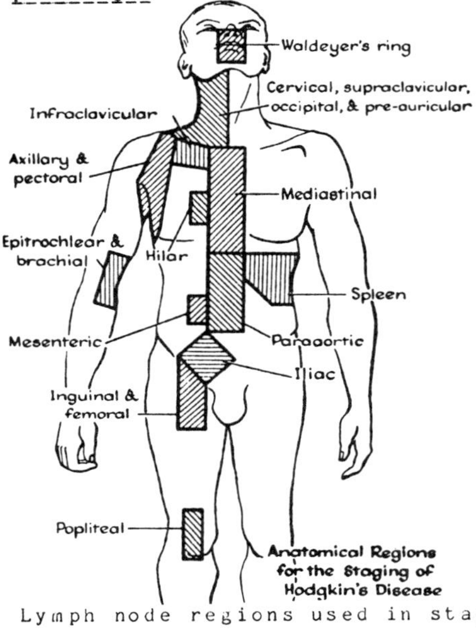

Figure 8.1. Lymph node regions used in staging (from Kaplan)

Stage I: Involvement of a single lymph node region (I) or of a single extralymphatic organ or site (IE).

Stage II: Involvement of two or more lymph node regions on the same side of the diaphragm (II) or localized involvement of an extralymphatic organ or site and of one or more lymph node regions on the same side of the diaphragm (IIE).

Stage III: Involvement of lymph node regions on both sides of the diaphragm (III), which may also be accompanied by localized involvement of extralymphatic organ or site (IIIE) or by involvement of the spleen (IIS) or both (IIIS-E). (Division of Stage III into IIIA1 and IIIA2 categories is addressed below).

Stage IV: Diffuse or disseminated involvement of one or more extralymphatic organs or tissues with or without associated lymph node enlargement. The reason for classifying the patient stage IV is identified by symbols:

N-Lymph nodes	S-Spleen
H-Liver	L-Lung
M-Marrow	O-Bone
P-Pleura	D-Skin

Systemic Symptoms

A: None present

B: Any or all of these:

1. Unexplained weight loss > 10% of body weight in six months prior to admission.
2. Unexplained fever with temperatures > 38°C.
3. Night sweats.

WORK-UP

In addition to a detailed history, with attention to B symptoms and careful physical examination with attention to all lymph node sites, the following work-up is required for clinical staging (CS) evaluation: Surgical biopsy, radiologic studies (chest x-ray, IVP, lymphangiogram, skeletal survey), laboratory studies (CBC with sed rate, alkaline phosphatase, BUN, SGOT, SGPT).

Pathologic Staging (PS) Evaluation: Involvement found at laparotomy or by any further removal of tissue for histologic examination other than that taken for the original diagnosis.

Specific Evaluation Studies and Procedures

1. Whole Lung Tomograms (to determine lung involvement): If mediastinal involvement is present on chest x-ray, there is a 20% likelihood of hilar involvement. Also, with hilar involvement has an important implication for radiation treatment planning since the ipsilateral lung is then at risk for involvement.

A CT scan of the thorax may supplement tomograms, since it is more sensitive in detecting pericardial and internal mammary node abnormalities which may be present with mediastinal disease, and in detecting lung disease when hilar nodes are positive. CT information may therefore result in more modification of the radiation fields than information obtained from tomography.

2. Bone Marrow Biopsy: The yield is low with Stage IA and IIA disease. Marrow biopsy is recommended:

a. In a patient with unexplained anemia.
b. In a patient with elevated alkaline phosphatase.
c. Stages III and IV disease or B symptoms.
d. X-ray or bone scan evidence of bone disease.

3. Abdominal and Pelvic CT Scan: A CT scan may be of value to complement the lymphangiogram, since a lower extremity lymphangiogram does not opacify internal iliac, hypogastric, mesenteric or presacral nodes. Upper abdominal lymph nodes (above L-2) are not reproducibly opacified well enough to allow accurate interpretation. The lymphangiogram does aid in field shaping and may be useful in follow-up.

4. Staging Laparotomy: A staging laparotomy is a diagnostic procedure used to obtain information about the extent of disease in the abdominal cavity. Surgical morbidity should be minimal. The procedure may upstage over 25 to 30% of patients and downstage 10%. A

significant determination gained from laparotomy and splenectomy is the presence or absence of splenic involvement, which is difficult to determine from a clinical basis alone. In addition, splenectomy allows reduction in the radiation field which may avoid radiation of much of the stomach, left lower lobe of the left lung, left kidney, and some small bowel. Laparotomy must be done with an adequate incision and should include:

a. Detailed abdominal inspection and palpation.
b. Splenectomy with metallic clips placed on the splenic pedicle for subsequent radiotherapeutic reference. Postsurgical pathologic analysis of the spleen includes gross examination, fixation, and resection in 1/2 cm slices.
c. Biopsies of each lobe of the liver (wedge and needle).
d. Nodal biopsies (para-aortic, iliac, splenic hilar, celiac, porta hepatis and mesentery). Suspicious nodes seen at laparotomy or previously suggested by lymphangiogram should also be biopsied and clipped. An intraoperative radiograph should be obtained to establish the position of clipped suspicious nodes.
e. Oophoropexy with midline placement and radioopaque clips.

Laparotomy should not be a routine procedure for all Hodgkin's disease patients but should be performed only on patients where the results may change the treatment plan. For example, a laparotomy may be avoided in patients with:

a. Clinical Stage IIIB or IV (it would be likely that treatment would consist of chemotherapy only initially).
b. Clinical Stage IA with high cervical nodes, and clinical Stage IA with mediastinal disease only. Avoidance of a laparotomy in these patients is debatable. One approach recommends a blind left scalene biopsy (unless thoracic duct drains to the right) if negative, laparotomy can be avoided; if positive, the patient goes on to laparotomy.

c. Clinical Stage I and IIA with a large mediastinal mass if combined therapy is planned (See below).
d. Children under the age of 10 are at a high risk for life threatening infections, especially with pneumococcal organisms in the first 18 months post-splenectomy. Thus, one must be highly selective performing splenectomy in this age group. Pneumococcal vaccine should be administered preoperatively and prophylactic antibiotics postoperatively.

As we improve our diagnostic and therapeutic capabilities, the indications for laparotomy will no doubt change.

TREATMENT AND RESULTS

The radiotherapy of Hodgkin's disease should be done in a radiation therapy department meeting several basic requirements.

1. Megavoltage equipment, preferably a linear accelerator of 4-6 MeV, so that large fields with shorter treatment times and sharper beam edges can be obtained compared to cobalt radiation.
2. Customized alloy block capabilities to protect normal tissues.
3. Computerized dosimetric planning which will establish the dose distribution throughout the treatment field.

The technique of treatment is highly important:

Fields are usually treated parallel opposed with equal weighting (i.e. half from the front and half from the back). Daily doses are usually 180 to 200 rad/day to a total dose of 3600-4400 rad. Typically, 3600 rad is given to clinically negative nodes, 4000 rad to clinically positive nodal areas and occasionally 4400 rad to areas of persistant bulky adenopathy.

Specific fields, which attempt to treat nodes in one contiguous treatment volume include:

Mantle: Mediastinal, hilar, cervical, axillary, supraclavicular and infraclavicular nodes.

Mini-Mantle: Same as mantle without mediastinal or hilar nodes.
Extended Mantle: Mantle including para-aortic nodes to L3 or L4. Increased morbidity over mantle and not used much.
Inverted Y: Spleen or splenic pedicle, para-aortic, iliac and femoral nodes.
Pelvis: Common and external iliacs, inguinal and femoral nodes.
Para-aortic and Splenic Pedicle: Para-aortic nodes (to approximately L4), splenic pedicle.
Waldeyer's Ring: Rarely used to treat Waldeyer's nodes (base of tongue, tonsil and nasopharynx). If high cervical nodes are involved, treatment of ipsilateral pre-auricular nodes is recommended.

These specific fields may be treated sequentially (usually to allow bone marrow recovery) and are referred to as:

Total Nodal Irradiation: Mantle and inverted Y, or mantle, para-aortic/splenic pedicle, pelvis.
Subtotal Nodal Irradiation: Mantle and para-aortic/splenic pedicle.

Radiotherapeutic techniques must take into account the details of the disease extent. The various options for each disease presentation are beyond the scope of this book. It may be worthwhile to review common presentations and general treatment policy.

EARLY DISEASE (Stage I, II)

Mantle and para-aortic/splenic pedicle irradiation is the preferred treatment for patients with early Hodgkin's disease. Results of treatment are excellent with 75-85% five year relapse-free survival. Salvage chemotherapy is effective in the majority of patients with recurrent disease so that overall survival rates are more than 90%. Subdiaphragmatic presentation is far less common but results of radiation therapy alone are good.

A supradiaphragmatic presentation of special interest includes patients with large mediastinal masses (greater than one-third of the maximum thoracic diameter or greater than 6 cm on a standing PA film). These patients have a somewhat higher relapse rate following radiation alone. In addition, they may not be candidates for initial staging laparotomy or lymphangiogram due to airway compromise even if not apparent on x-ray. One management approach is to treat a mantle field which may include the whole affected lung(s) at 150 rad/day to 1500 rad. After a two week treatment break, if tumor shrinkage has occurred, the alloy blocks are recut and radiation continued to 4000 rad. The blocks are frequently recut to conform to the tumor shrinkage. Laparotomy can be performed after mantle irradiation is completed. If no significant tumor shrinkage occurs at 1500 rad, chemotherapy may be used to avoid exceeding lung tolerance to radiation. Another approach is to use chemotherapy initially, using radiation later to areas of prior bulk disease to consolidate treatment.

Chemotherapy for early stage Hodgkins disease (I, IIA) has been advocated and used in a small number of patients. Durable remissions may not be as successfully obtained as with radiotherapy and morbidity (particularly sterility) is greater. However, initial chemotherapy in conjunction with low dose radiation has been found to be quite successful in pediatric Hodgkin's disease. In pre-pubertal children, radiation may result in growth problems; combined modality treatment has been used with success though sterility is a lasting problem.

ADVANCED DISEASE (Stage III, Stage IV)

The development of effective combination chemotherapy has dramatically improved the cure rate in advanced Hodgkin's disease over the past two decades. Radiotherapy still has an important and curative role in selected patients with stage IIIA disease as described below. Additionally, radiotherapy may be a useful adjunct to chemotherapy in maintaining long-term remissions. Radiotherapy is not frequently successful in salvaging chemotherapy failure.

Stage IIIA disease may be treated with radiotherapy alone but the relapse rate may be as high as 50%. There is some indication that there may be two (or more) prognostic subgroups: Stage IIIA1 where disease is limited to the upper abdomen, involving spleen, splenic hilum, celiac or portal nodes; and IIIA2, where disease is located in the para-aortic, iliac or mesenteric nodes. In patients treated with radiation, those with Stage IIIA1 disease do better than those with Stage IIIA2 disease. Patients with Stage IIIA2 disease tend to fail in the liver and elsewhere. Presently, most patients with Stage IIIA2 disease are treated with chemotherapy. Patients with IIIA disease with multiple sites (>5) of involvement or with 5 or more splenic nodules may benefit from systemic chemotherapy in addition to radiation.

Stage IIIB and IV disease can be treated successfully with combination chemotherapy. Chemotherapy with MOPP (nitrogen mustard, vincristine, procarbazine and prednisone) has been the standard treatment for most advanced Hodgkin's disease. Eighty percent of patients treated with MOPP are complete responders with 68% of these remaining disease-free at five years. Thus, 55% of patients remain in long-term remission at five years. Other treatment regimens are being investigated to improve these results as well as to decrease the toxicity. One approach is the use of sequential non-cross resistant chemotherapy, e.g. MOPP and ABVD (adriamycin, bleomycin, velban and DTIC). Another avenue of investigation is the use of low-dose radiotherapy (1500-2000 rad) to areas of pretreatment clinical involvement following complete response to chemotherapy in an attempt to prolong the disease-free survival.

Table 8.1 indicates survival and relapse-free survival with present treatment techniques.

Table 8.1
Results of Treatment for Hodgkin's Disease

STAGE	INITIAL TREATMENT	5 YEAR RELAPSE-FREE SURVIVAL (%)	5 YEAR* SURVIVAL (%)
IA, IIA	RADIATION	75-90	90-95
IB, IIB	RADIATION	70-85	90
IIIA	RADIATION	50-75	80
IIIA1	RADIATION	75	80-95
IIIA2	RADIATION	25	50-65
IIIA	CHEMOTHERAPY	50-90	50-90
IIIB, IV	CHEMOTHERAPY	40-50	50-60

*Includes chemotherapy for salvage in Stage I,II, III_A and includes combined modality results in advanced disease.

MORBIDITY (Discussion limited to radiotherapy morbidity)

Most radiation complications are related to mantle irradiation. Special blocks are used when appropriate to limit the dose to the larynx, cardiac apex, spinal cord, and humeral heads.

Acute Reactions

Skin reactions are transient and usually mild to moderate. Commonly dry desquamation, erythema and hyperpigmentation are seen but occasionally focal areas of moist desquamation may be noted.

Xerostomia usually develops during radiation and usually is mild and transient, unlike that seen with high dose radiation given for cancers arising in head and neck sites.

Odynophagia of mild, transient nature may occur during the second or third week of mantle irradiation and responds to topical anesthetics (e.g. Oxaine-M) or analgesics and subsides after completion of mantle irradiation.

Nausea may occur early in the course of treatment and may be controlled with antiemetics or cannabinoids.

Hair loss is temporary. It occurs in the occipital region as well as the axillae and irradiated chest regions.

Myelosuppression occurs when significant bone marrow is irradiated as in most extended fields. It is usually mild and transient. For example, following mantle irradiation an approximate 2-3 week treatment break is given to allow recovery from mild leukopenia and thrombocytopenia prior to irradiating infradiaphragmatic fields. When total nodal irradiation is used or when irradiation follows chemotherapy, myelosuppression may be severe and blood counts must be closely monitored.

Chronic Reactions

Pneumonitis: Symptomatic pneumonits is seen in 2-5% of patients treated with mantle fields.

Carditis: Clinically relevant pericarditis occurs in less than 3% of patients. Nonconstrictive "acute" pericarditis may appear weeks to years following radiation. The most common manifestation is a pericardial effusion with fever, tachycardia, substernal pain and friction rub. It is important to evaluate thyroid function to rule out hypothyroidism as an alternate etiology. The course is usually self-limiting but about half the patients may develop constrictive pericarditis. Doses of over 3000 rad to the whole heart may result in a high incidence of pericarditis (50%). When whole heart irradiation is required, cardiac apical blocks should be used at a dose of 1500 to 2000 rad. Unequal field weighting which may result in delivery of high doses of radiation to the heart should be avoided. Constrictive pericarditis occurs 6 months to years following radiation, and may or may not be preceded by "acute" pericarditis. Treatment depends on severity. The production of myocardiopathy or coronary artery disease by radiation is rare.

Infertility: Transient oligospermia or ovarian dysfunction is seen whenever pelvic lymph nodes are treated, due to scattered radiation to the testicles or ovary. In males, with scrotal shielding, the testicular dose can be kept below 100 rad and permanent oligospermia should be rare. In females, with midline oophoropexy and a central pelvic block of 10HVL, the dose to the ovaries is minimal. Transient menstrual irregularities are common with recovery the rule, but 20% or less of females treated with inverted Y fields may develop persistent menstrual irregularities and infertility.

Lhermitte's Sign: This is a transient complication seen in about 15% of patients undergoing mantle irradiation and consists of numbness, tingling or "electric" sensations produced with head flexion. It is not associated with any subsequent neurologic problems when standard radiation doses have been administered.

Hypothyroidism: Clinical hypothyroidism may develop in less than 10% of patients following mantle irradiation. Its incidence may be higher in patients who have undergone a lymphangiogram for staging. Chemical thyroid dysfunction, particularly elevated TSH, is seen more frequently. All patients should have baseline T3, T4 and TSH levels as well as follow-up levels so that thyroid dysfunction can be corrected. It is not clear if one should administer treatment with only TSH elevation or wait for possible hypothyrodism to develop.

Leukemia: Leukemia may develop following combined radiotherpy and chemotherapy treatment for Hodgkin's disease. Refractory, fatal ANLL develops in 7-10% of patients treated successfully with chemotherapy alone or chemotherapy in combination with radiation. It arises several years following completion of treatment.

Others: Bone growth arrest (seen in children).

NON-HODGKIN'S LYMPHOMA

OVERVIEW

This group of diseases is unlike Hodgkin's disease in pathology, clinical features, or response to treatment. Non-Hodgkin's lymphomas share the same Ann Arbor staging system with Hodgkin's disease but, although they frequently respond quite well to radiotherapy or chemotherapy, they are much less curable.

PATHOLOGY

The Rappaport system is the most widely used pathologic classification system. It is based on the architectural pattern (nodular or diffuse) and the cell type (well differentiated lymphocytic, poorly differentiated lymphocytic, histiocytic, or mixed). Although this system is clinically useful, there have been objections to it, since it does not correctly describe the cells of origin or incorporate current immunologic concepts (among others).

A Working Formulation has been proposed to address these issues. Lymphomas are divided into three grades which reflect the clinical behavior. Each grade has three or four subtypes with distinctly different behavior. A translation is offered in Table 8.2.

About half of patients present with nodular lymphoma. However, a substantial number of patients with nodular lymphoma will evolve to a diffuse pattern as part of the natural history of their disease. It is also likely that the small indolent lymphocytes comprising most nodular lymphomas gradually may evolve to the large transformed lymphocytes of histiocytic lymphomas. The greater tendency of the small untransformed lymphocyte to migrate in the circulation correlates with the generally widespread presentation of lymphocytic lymphomas as opposed to the more frequently localized presentation of histiocytic lymphomas.

Table 8.2
Comparison of Rappaport Classification and Working Formulation

WORKING FORMULATION	RAPPAPORT EQUIVALENT*
LOW GRADE	
Small Lymphocytic	DLWD
Follicular, predominantly small cell, cleaved	NLPD
Follicular, mixed small cell, cleaved, and large cell	NM
INTERMEDIATE GRADE	
Follicular, predominantly large cell	NH
Diffuse, small cleaved cell	DLPD
Diffuse, mixed small and large cell	DM
Diffuse, large cell	DH
HIGH GRADE	
Large cell, immunoblastic	DH
Lymphoblastic	LB
Small non-cleaved cell	DU

*Where for Rappaport Classsification:
Architecture: D=diffuse N=nodular

Cell Type: LWD=lymphocytic well differentiated
LPD=lymphocytic poorly differentiated
H=histiocytic
M=mixed lymphocytic & histologic
U=undifferentiated
LB=lymphoblastic

CLINICAL FEATURES

The median age at diagnosis is 50-60 years. Most non-Hodgkin's lymphomas are derived from B cells or null cells (except for lymphoblastic lymphoma). They are seldom localized (less than 10%) infrequently involve the mediastinum (less than 20%), and are more likely to involve peripheral nodal regions (e.g. epitrochlear, Waldeyer's) and mesenteric nodes than Hodgkin's disease. Bone marrow and liver involvement are common, particularly with nodular lymphomas. Systemic symptoms are less frequent in non-Hodgkin's than in Hodgkin's lymphoma, and do not seem to be important prognostically.

The non-Hodgkin's lymphomas can be grouped into favorable, "indolent" histologies (NLWD, DLWD, NLPD, NM) and unfavorable, "aggressive" histologies (DH, DLPD, DM). The patients with favorable histologies usually present with slowly progressive lymphadenopathy, and over 90% will have advanced Stage III or IV disease. Patients with unfavorable histologies usually present with rapidly progressive lymphadenopathy but 30-45% may have Stage I or II disease.

Lymphoblastic lymphoma: This lymphoma is usually of T-cell origin and typically presents as a mediastinal mass in a young male. Hematologic, bone marrow and central nervous system involvement are often present.

Burkitt's lymphoma: This B cell lymphoma is commonly seen in children. Although in African children it usually presents as a mass in the maxilla or jaw, in Americans it commonly presents with extensive intra-abdominal disease. Epstein-Barr virus antigen can be frequently identified in the African variety, much less so in the American variety. The disease is very aggressive with an estimated doubling time of just two days.

STAGING

Same as Hodgkin's disease (See above). The Ann Arbor system is used.

WORK-UP

In addition to history and physical, primary evaluation should include:

Radiologic studies: (chest x-ray, lymphangiogram and/or abdominal CT scan), Laboratory studies (CBC, sed rate, SGOT, SGPT, alkaline phosphatase, BUN, creatinine, uric acid).

Bone marrow biopsy. Bilateral iliac crest biopsies need to be performed since sampling error with a single biopsy can be 10-15% in favorable lymphomas.

Others: IVP, when bulky retroperitoneal adenopathy is present. Upper G.I. with small bowel follow through if Waldeyer's ring is involved, since there may be associated involvement in 10% of patients. Liver biopsy in Stage III patients, if hepatic involvement will change therapy. CSF evaluation in pediatric undifferentiated and lymphoblastic lymphomas. Direct Coomb's should be obtained particularly in patients with anemia, since auto-immune hemolytic anemia may occur with non-Hodgkin's lymphoma.

Staging laparotomy is not indicated in most cases since the results rarely affect treatment decision. In particular, laparotomy can usually be avoided since the procedures outlined above, particular lymphangiogram plus or minus CT scan, bone marrow biopsy and liver biopsy are quite accurate in staging with only approximately 10% false negatives.

TREATMENT AND RESULTS

General

Radiotherapy has a curative potential in some patients with non-Hodgkin's lymphoma, in particular those with early disease. A high degree of local control (>90%) can be obtained with doses of 2500 to 3500 rad in all but diffuse histiocytic lymphoma. With diffuse histiocytic lymphoma most radiotherapists use higher doses (4500-5000 rad) for local control.

Single agent and combination chemotherapy have been used extensively in the treatment for non-Hodgkin's lymphoma. Combination chemotherapy regimens are numerous; several well known regimens include MOPP, C-MOPP (cytoxan, vincristine, procarbaine, prednisone), BACOP (bleomycin, doxorubicin, cytoxan, vincristine, prednisone) and CHOP (cytoxan, doxorubicin, vincristine, prednisone). Combination chemotherapy claims a curative potentitial in patients with advanced stage diffuse histiocytic lymphoma.

Combined modality approaches using combination chemotherapy along with involved field or extended field radiation have not yet demonstrated superior results. Investigations to identify subgroups of patients where this approach may be effective are ongoing.

EARLY DISEASE (Stage I and Stage II)

Overall, more than 60% of patients with localized disease (Stage I and contiguous Stage II) or localized extranodal lymphoma (Stage IE) can be cured with radiotherapy alone. There is no obvious survival advantage between using small, intermediate or large radiation fields.

Favorable Histologies: The infrequent occurence of early stage favorable histology lymphoma and its indolent natural history require long periods of observation before sufficient data can be accumulated regarding treatment efficacy. Radiotherapy has traditionally been the treatment of choice and has a proven efficacy. Freedom from relapse following radiation diminishes from over 60% at five years to about 50% at ten years. Relapse usually occurs in contiguous or non-contiguous nodal sites when less than total nodal radiation is given, as opposed to extralymphatic relapse when total nodal radiation is given. There is a flattening of the relapse curve suggesting a cure rate of about 50%.

Unfavorable Histologies: Early stage unfavorable histology lymphoma, though mostly all diffuse histiocytic, represents a heterogeneous group. Factors which may influence treatment outcome include site of disease presentation, nodal versus extranodal disease, bulk of disease, age of the patient as well as clinical versus pathologic staging. Overall, radiotherapy is the treatment of choice, though the addition of chemotherapy may be of value in the treatment of early stage diffuse histiocytic lymphoma. The majority of patients presenting with gastric, bone or head and neck involvement can be cured with radiation whereas CNS presentation is rarely curable. In general, extranodal involvement and stage I disease are associated with better survival. Failure is less frequent with radiotherapy alone in patients with less than 4 sites of involvement or disease less than 2.5 cm size. Patients under age 60 with bulky (> 2.5 cm) tumors may do better than patients over age 60. Laparotomy may identify abdominal involvement in a small proportion of localized unfavorable lymphomas, so clinical and pathologic staging are not entirely equivalent. The use of chemotherapy alone and combined modality treatment are being investigated for stage I and II malignant lymphoma of unfavorable histology (particularly DHL).

ADVANCED DISEASE (Stage III, Stage IV)

Favorable Histology: Treatment approaches for advanced stage indolent disease are palliative only. Asymptomatic patients may be followed for a median of three years before treatment is needed for palliation. Their overall median survival is ten years. Symptomatic patients are responsive to single alkylating agents (50-60% complete response), combination chemotherapy (70% complete response) and whole body irradiation (60% complete response). Since treatment is palliative, it is important that it is not continued indefinitely but rather stopped after complete remission is documented. As one form of treatment, whole body irradiation can be administered as 15 rad twice weekly to a dose of 75 rad followed by a treatment break to allow for recovery in platelet count then repeating the irradiation to a total dose of 150 rad.

Unfavorable Histology: Systemic combination chemotherapy claims a curative potential for patients with stage III and IV diffuse histiocytic lymphoma. Complete response rates of 40-60% are reported with most being sustained through 3-5 years. Combined modality results using chemotherapy and consolidative radiotherapy may result in improved survival in patients with stage III disease.

OTHERS

Burkitt's Lymphoma: Treatment is primarily with systemic chemotherapy. Surgery may be useful in debulking large intra-abdominal disease. Radiotherapy is often used in prophylactic cranial treatment and may be useful in consolidating treatment to areas of bulk disease. It is very important that patients are hydrated and allopurinol is administered prior to chemotherapy initiation since rapid response could result in uric acid nephropathy and metabolic imbalance, particularly hyperkalemia.

Lymphoblastic Lymphoma: This lymphoma should be treated as a T-cell leukemia with multi-agent chemotherapy, intrathecal methotrexate and cranial irradiation.

MORBIDITY

Treatment morbidity of non-Hodgkin's lymphomas is highly dependent on the region irradiated. The reader is referred to the morbidity section of Hodgkin's disease for a general discussion of morbidity of irradiation.

SOLITARY PLASMACYTOMA

Solitary plasma cell tumors represent less than 10% of myelomas. Those occurring in bone commonly represent an early stage of myeloma since the vast majority progress to multiple myeloma if follow-up is long enough. In contrast, solitary extramedullary plasmacytomas often are truly localized and can be cured in nearly 80% of patients when localized radiation therapy of 4500-5500 rad is given.

MULTIPLE MYELOMA

Local radiation therapy (2000-4000 rad) can be effective in palliating bone pain.

LEUKEMIAS

The treatment of leukemia involves radiotherapy in several different roles.

ACUTE LEUKEMIA

Acute Lymphocytic Leukemia (ALL)

Prophylactic cranial irradiation: Patients with initial white counts greater than 50,000 or age less than 2 or greater than 7 are considered high risk candidates for relapse, including CNS relapse. Other factors associated with a poorer prognosis include T-cell and Ph chromosome (+) ALL, race (blacks do worse) and lymphoma syndrome (lymphadenopathy ± splenomegaly). After completion of induction chemotherapy, 1800 rad cranial irradiation and intrathecal methotrexate are administered to prevent CNS relapse in high risk patients. Without prophylactic treatment at least 50% of patients who are in bone marrow remission post induction will have relapse in the central nervous system. Radiation is given to the whole cranium, retro-orbital area and spine to the level of C_2. Since careful immobilization is needed during treatment, sedation is sometimes required.

Controversy exists as to whether prophylactic cranial irradiation produces deleterious effects on brain development. The use of intermittent systemic methotrexate during maintenance is not as effective as radiation in cranial prophylaxis but may offer better protection against systemic relapse in standard risk patients.

Testicular Radiation: Radiation doses of 1800 to 2400 rad have been used to treat testicular relapse. Patients undergo routine testicular biopsy at two years, prior to discontinuing maintenance chemotherapy. If biopsy is microscopically positive, the testicles are irradiated and chemotherapy is continued but prognosis is still relatively good. Patients with grossly positive testicular relapse have a very poor prognosis. Testicular irradiation and reinduction chemotherapy are required and are not frequently successful.

Acute Non-Lymphocytic Leukemia (ANLL)

Prophylactic cranial irradiation may be of value in preventing CNS relapse.

Whole body irradiation to fractionated doses of approximately 1000 rad, e.g. 333 rad x 3 along with cyclophosphamide are employed to induce marrow aplasia and deter graft versus host reactions prior to bone marrow transplant.

CHRONIC LEUKEMIAS

Chronic Lymphocytic Leukemia (CLL)

Whole body irradiation (as an alternative to alkylating agents) with low fraction sizes of 15 rad to doses of 75-150 rad may be used in the treatment of chronic lymphocytic leukemia. Approximately one-third of patients undergo a complete remisson. The median survival of CLL patients treated with total body irradiation is nearly 5 years.

Chronic Myelogenous Leukemia (CML)

CML is usually treated with alkylating agents. Splenic irradiation has been used as an alternative to drugs to treat splenomegaly, particularly in CML. Often an abscopal effect (i.e. a response in tissues other than those irradiated) is seen in circulating blood elements. Several daily doses of 25 to 50 rad may be sufficient to reduce splenomegaly but doses must remain low to avoid inducing pancytopenia. During the blastic phase radiation is usually of little value.

REFERENCES

1. Coltman CA, Jr (ed). Hodgkin's disease. Semin Oncol 7:91, 1980.
2. DeVita V et al: Curability of advanced Hodgkin's disease with chemotherapy. Ann Int Med 92:587-595, 1980.
3. Durant J et al: BCNU, velban, cyclophosphamide, procarbazine and prednisone (BCVPP) in advanced Hodgkin's disease. Cancer 42:2101-2110, 1978.
4. Hellman S, Mauch P, Goodman RL et al: The place of radiation therapy in the treatment of Hodgkin's disease. Cancer 42:971-978, 1978.
5. Hoppe RT et al: Prognostic factors in pathologic stage IIIA Hodgkin's disease. Cancer 46:1240-1246, 1980.

6. Kinsella T et al: Late effects of radiation therapy in the treatment of Hodgkin's disease. Canc Treat Rept 66:991-1001, 1982.
7. Krikorian JG et al: Hodgkin's disease, stages I & II occuring below the diaphragm. Cancer 43:1866-1871, 1979.
8. Stein RS et al: Anatomic substages of stage III_A Hodgkin's disease. Ann Int Med 92:159-165, 1980.
9. Bitran JD et al: Survival of patients with localized histiocytic lymphoma. Cancer 39:342-346, 1977.
10. Calsanillas F et al: Mangement with chemotherapy only of stage I & II malignant lymphoma of aggressive histologic types. Cancer 46:2356-2359, 1980.
11. Fisher RI et al: Prognostic factors for advanced diffuse histiocytic lymphoma following treatment with combined chemotherapy. Am J Med 63:177-182, 1977.
12. Glatstein E et al: Combined modality therapy in malignant lymphoma. Canc Treat Rept 61:1199-1207, 1977.
13. Levitt S et al: Curative radiotherapy for localized diffuse histiocytic lymphoma. Canc Treat Rept 64:175-177, 1980.
14. Montardini S et al: Improved 5-year survival after combined radiotherapy - chemotherapy for stage I-II non-Hodgkin's lymphoma. I J Rad Bio Phys 16:125-134, 1980.
15. Toonkel L et al: Laparotomy staged I & II non-Hodgkin's lymphoma cancer. Cancer 45:249-260, 1980.

Chapter 9

Lung Cancer Mesothelioma and Thymoma

LUNG CANCER

OVERVIEW

There is presently an epidemic of carcinoma of the lung in the United States with an estimated 135,000 new cases in 1983 with approximately 117,000 deaths, accounting for 25% of all cancer deaths. The majority of patients present with distant metastatic disease or locally advanced tumor. Of the 30% of cases that present with operable disease, only half will be resectable at surgery. There is another subgroup of patients who have resectable disease but are medically inoperable due to advanced cardiopulmonary disease. Thus, most patients with lung cancer will require radiotherapeutic intervention sometime during their course either as curative therapy for inoperable or locally advanced cancer or for palliation of symptoms related to intrathoracic disease or distant metastases.

PATHOLOGY

The World Health Organization (WHO) published its most recent lung classification in 1981 recognizing five major histologic types. These are listed in Table 9.1 along with their approximate frequency.

Table 9.1
WHO Lung Cancer Classification 1981

Histology	Frequency
Squamous cell carcinoma	35%
Small cell carcinoma	20-25%
Adenocarcinoma	25-35%
Large cell carcinoma	15%
Adenosquamous carcinoma	1-3%

In recent decades there has been a significant decrease in the incidence of squamous cell carcinoma along with a rise in the incidence of adenocarcinoma. In one recently reported series, adenocarcinoma was the most common histologic type of lung cancer. Bronchioalveolar carcinoma is a relatively rare cancer classified along with adenocarcinomas. The biologic behavior of small cell carcinoma is sufficiently different from the other histologic types, that this tumor type will be discussed separately below. Another pathologic entity that deserves mention is the mixed small cell-large cell carcinoma, which appears to have the same metastatic pattern as small cell carcinoma but the objective response rate to chemotherapy is less, as is the median survival.

CLINICAL FEATURES

Lung cancer is still a relatively rare disease in non-smokers. There is a "dose-response" effect appparent among smokers with the incidence increasing with the number of packs consumed per day. Industrial pollutants including asbestos, nickel, arsenic, uranium and chloromethyl ether have been linked with the development of bronchogenic carcinomas. The male to female ratio is 4:1 with the incidence in females increasing dramatically. The peak incidence is age 50-60 years.

Lung cancers often reach large sizes before symptoms develop. Locally they can manifest with symptoms such as cough, hemoptysis, stridor, change in a chronic cough, dyspnea, chest pain, pleural effusion, pneumonitis or hoarseness. Other distinct manifestations of loco-regional spread include the superior vena caval syndrome, commonly seen with right upper lobe lesions and Pancoast syndrome due to superior sulcus tumors extending superiorly into the brachial plexus, ribs and sympathetic chain. Often times, symptoms related to metastatic disease involving the central nervous system or the skeleton are the first clues of a bronchogenic carcinoma. Paraneoplastic syndromes are well described and including Cushing's syndrome, carcinoid syndrome, syndrome of inappropriate ADH secretion, hyercalcemia, Eaton-Lamberts' syndrome, cerebellar degeneration, hypertrophic pulmonary osteoarthropathy and dermatomyositis.

STAGING

The American Joint Committee's TNM system is widely accepted for non-small cell lung cancers.

TNM Classification

Primary Tumor (T)

- TX Tumor proven by the presence of malignant cells in bronchopulmonary secretions but not visualized roentgenographically or bronchoscopically; or any tumor that cannot be assessed.
- T0 No evidence of primary tumor
- TIS Carcinoma in situ
- T1 Tumor 3.0 cm or less in greatest diameter, or a tumor of any size that either invades the visceral pleura or has associated atelectasis or obstructive pneumonitis extending to the hilar region. At bronchoscopy, the proximal extent of demonstrable tumor must be within a lobal bronchus or at least 2.0 cm distal to the carina. Any associated atelectasis or obstructive pneumonitis must involve less than an entire lung and there must be no pleural effusion.
- T2 Tumor 3.0 cm or greater or a tumor of any size that either invades visceral pleura or has associated atelectasis or obstructive pneumonitis extending to hila. Proximal extent of tumor must be in a lobar bronchus or 2.0 cm distal to the carina. No pleural effusion. Atelectasis or obstructive pneumonitis must not involve an entire lung.
- T3 Direct extension into an adjacent structure; or tumor involving a main bronchus less than 2.0 cm from carina; or any tumor with atelectasis or obstructive pneumonitis involving an entire lung or a pleural effusion.

Nodal Involvement (N)

- N0 No demonstrable metastasis to regional lymph nodes
- N1 Metastasis to lymph nodes in the peribronchial or the ipsilateral hilar region, or both, including direct extension
- N2 Metastasis to lymph nodes in the mediastinum

Distant Metastasis (M)

MX Not assessed
M0 No (known) distant metastasis
M1 Distant metastasis present

Stage Group

Occult Carcinoma
TX N0 M0
Stage I
TIS N0 M0
T1 N0 M0
T1 N1 M0
T2 N0 M0
Stage II
T2 N1 M0
Stage III
T3; any N or M
N2; any T or M
M1; any T or N

The VA Lung Study Group's staging system for small cell cancer:

1. Limited disease: Tumor confined to one hemithorax with or without ipsilateral supraclavicular adenopathy.
2. Extensive disease: Tumor has spread beyond the hemithorax or pleural effusion present with positive cytology.

WORK-UP

Once a diagnosis of bronchogenic carcinoma is suspected on the basis of symptomatology and routine chest radiography, it is highly desirable to establish a tissue diagnosis in all cases because the treatment of small cell carcinoma involves the use of systemic chemotherapy, which is only of minimal effectiveness for the other cell types. Diagnosis can be established with serial sputum collections for cytology, bronchoscopy for biopsy and cytologic brushings of endobronchial tumors, transthoracic needle aspiration for peripheral lesions, mediastinoscopy, mediastinotomy (Chamberlain procedure), scalene node biopsy and thoracotomy. The remainder of the staging work-up should be tailored to the histologic type, results of the physical and neurologic examinations, results of the chemical profile, clinical symptoms and the operability status on medical grounds. Radionuclide liver/spleen scans, bone scans and brain scans have low yields in the absence of clinical symptomatology or abnormalities of the chemical profile.

CT scanning of the chest still must prove itself as a means of determining the extent of mediastinal involvement. Early studies using first generation CT scanners disclosed an unacceptable number of false negative scans when compared to mediastinoscopy (20%). Nevertheless, the technique does provide the radiation therapist with valuable information regarding the spatial relationships of the tumor and mediastinal nodes to vital structures such as the spinal cord and heart. When combined with computer-assisted treatment planning, the CT scan allows the radiation therapist to optimize dose delivery to sites of disease.

Gallium scanning is advocated as an accurate way of staging lung cancer patients, although the method is not universally accepted. Bone marrow aspirate and biopsy should be performed in all patients with small cell cancer due to a 15-20% incidence of bone marrow involvement. Brain CT scans have a 6% yield in lung cancer patients with no neurologic symptoms or signs but their use in clinical staging must be considered investigational.

TREATMENT AND RESULTS

NON-SMALL CELL LUNG CANCER

The treatment of choice for lung cancer remains surgical intervention performing the minimum amount of surgery to accomplish total tumor removal. There is a significantly lower risk of local failure in patients with T1 and T2 tumors undergoing resection compared to those treated with radiation alone. The role of radiation therapy in the management of lung cancer can be divided into three categories: (1) definitive, (2) adjuvant and (3) palliative.

Definitive Radiation Therapy

Medically Inoperable Stage I and Stage II Disease: Some patients with early stage lung cancer are deemed unsuitable for thoracotomy because of medical problems such as severe cardiopulmonary disease. In selected patients with small tumor burdens (Stage I & II), cure can be achieved in up to 25% of patients with careful delivery of high doses of radiation therapy (not too dissimilar from the cure rate obtained with surgery). Many people argue that such patients should not be treated until they develop symptoms referrable to their malignant disease; however, this significant chance for a cure is forfeited by such a watch-and-wait policy. It has been our experience that when such patients are offered such therapy they embrace it wholeheartedly.

Advanced Unresectable Local-regional Disease (Stage III): This group of patients are found to be unresectable during the staging work-up or at the time of exploratory thoracotomy because of *local extension of tumor to the mediastinum or chest wall* or because of extensive *mediastinal nodal metastases*. In general, mediastinal nodal metastases are the harbinger of distant dissemination. Nevertheless, a small group of patients who have truly localized disease can be salvaged with aggressive thoracic irradiation. A recently completed Radiation Therapy Oncology Group (RTOG) study investigating four different dose-fractionation regimens showed that local control within the irradiated volume could be obtained in 55-63% of patients treated with doses ranging from 5000-6000 rad. Five year survival for this group ranges between 5-8%.

Adjuvant Radiation Therapy

Preoperative Radiotherapy: Radiation therapy given preoperatively to lung cancer patients has been shown to increase resectability but has had no major impact on survival compared with surgery alone in several randomized series. Doses have ranged between 3000 rad in 2 weeks and 4500 rad in 4 1/2 weeks. One non-randomized study showed a survival advantage to preoperative radiation therapy, but this experience has not been duplicated except in the case of superior sulcus tumors (Pancoast tumor).

Pancoast tumors are usually squamous cell carcinomas or adenocarcinomas arising in either pulmonary apex, locally eroding the upper thoracic ribs and extending to involve the brachial plexus and the cervical sympathetics. Traditional management has consisted of preoperative radiation therapy with doses ranging from 3000 rad over a two week period to 6000 rad over 6 weeks followed by maximal en bloc tumor resection including the removal of part of the involved vertebral bodies and chest wall. This has yielded five year survivals in the range of 35%. The approach at Memorial Sloan-Kettering Cancer Center has been similar, however, iodine-125 implants have been carried out for any residual tumor deposits. Recently, the Medical College of Wisconsin has reported a 24% five year survival in patients treated with high dose external beam radiotherapy alone. Pain relief was achieved in 86% of these patients.

Postoperative Radiotherapy: N0 (no nodal metastases): Radiation therapy has not been shown to increase survival in patients who have undergone curative resection for stage I disease. No postoperative radiation therapy is indicated in this group.

N1, N2 (hilar, mediastinal nodal metastases): Several retrospective reviews have shown a survival benefit to patients who have undergone "curative resections" and have been found to harbor hilar or mediastinal nodal metastases. Five year survivals of 30% can be achieved in patients receiving postoperative irradiation compared to about 2% for patients not receiving radiotherapy. There are conflicting reports about whether this benefit is restricted to only the squamous cell carcinoma histology. A prospective randomized trial investigating postoperative radiation therapy is presently being carried out by the European Organization for Research in the Treatment of Cancer (EORTC) (but note that this study also examines the role of chemoimmunotherapy as adjuvants).

Other: There are several other instances where a high risk for local recurrence exists and could conceivably be improved by postoperative irradiation.

These include patients with chest wall invasion, positive vascular or bronchial margins and tumor embolization into lymphatic channels.

Palliative Radiotherapy

As with many other sites, the palliative role of radiation therapy in lung cancer is unquestioned. Several studies have shown consistent relief of hemoptysis, chest pain and dyspnea in 60-80% of patients. Atelectasis is improved in 25% and hoarseness in 5%. The management of the superior vena caval syndrome is discussed in Chapter 16. Symptoms related to brain, bone or liver metastases can be significantly palliated with radiotherapy to these sites (See Chapter 17).

SMALL CELL LUNG CANCER

This histologic subtype is generally not amenable to surgery, although reports of cure by resection of small peripheral nodules are well documented. Small cell lung cancer is usually a systemic disease at the time of initial diagnosis. With careful staging up to 80% of patients can be shown to have extrathoracic disease, i.e. extensive stage at presentation.

Limited Stage Small Cell Lung Cancer

Untreated cases of limited stage small cell lung cancer have a median survival of approximately 12 weeks. Thoracic irradiation yields a complete response in a third of patients and partial response in another third, extending the median survival to 8 months with 11% of patients surviving two years. Combination chemotherapy alone consisting of cyclophosphamide, adriamycin and DTIC has produced a median survival of 10.6 months in patients with limited disease, superior to that achieved by radiation therapy alone. Several studies have investigated the use of consolidative irradiation "sandwiched" between courses of chemotherapy. Combined modality therapy has produced median survivals of up to 12 months and 36% two year survival for patients with limited stage disease.

Extensive Stage Small Cell Lung Cancer

Patients with extensive stage small cell carcinoma have metastatic disease which usually involves several sites. Untreated, the median survival is about six weeks. The mainstay of treatment is combination chemotherapy with complete response rates of up to 40% and total response rates greater than 90% reported. The median survival is approximately seven months with less than 5% of patients surviving two years. Consolidative radiotherapy of intrathoracic disease in patients obtaining complete or partial responses to chemotherapy should be considered since up to 80% of patients will eventually fail at the primary site.

Fifteen to 20% of patients with small cell carcinoma will develop brain metastases. Prophylactic brain irradiation (PBI) can reduce this incidence to less than 5%. All randomized studies have failed to show a survival benefit with the use of PBI. Most oncologists feel that PBI should be reserved for those small cell lung cancer patients who obtain complete responses to primary management.

Special Topics in the Treatment of Lung Cancer

Interstitial radiation therapy: Pioneering work done at Memorial Sloan-Kettering Cancer Center by Hilaris et al has shown the utility of intraoperative implantation of unresectable lung cancers with various encapsulated radioisotopes such as gold-198, radon-222 and iodine-125. Excellent local control in the range of 60-80% can be obtained. Overall, only 7% attained prolonged five year disease free survival, but a 33% disease-free five year survival was seen in patients with unresectable superior sulcus tumors. Such therapy can be combined with external beam irradiation given pre or postoperatively.

Large field irradiation: Hemibody irradiation has been studied as a form of "systemic treatment" in small cell carcinoma. A delay in the appearance of distant disease may be seen with hemibody irradiation but in general it does not have a significant impact on the disease. The toxicity may be prohibitive when large field irradiation is combined with chemotherapy.

Transbronchial brachytherapy: Endobronchial tumor masses can be implanted through a rigid bronchoscope or a flexible fiberoptic bronchoscope, again using encapsulated isotopes such as gold-198 or iodine-125. Patients must be carefully selected and are usually those who have failed surgery or external beam irradiation. Palliative benefit has been shown, especially when this technique is coupled with external beam irradiation. Optimal placement of brachytherapy sources is difficult.

MORBIDITY

Acute Reaction

Esophagitis: The esophagus is the most sensitive organ to react acutely to external beam thoracic irradiation. Some dysphagia will develop usually in the third week of treatment. This can be palliated by the use of local anesthetic and/or antacids, such as viscous xylocaine. Occasionally, the dysphagia will be due to candida infection and this will respond to the use of appropriate antifungal medications such as nystatin or ketoconazole (Nizoral). Occasionally, a treatment break will need to be imposed. The use of a planned treatment break, employed in a "split course" technique, allows healing of the esophageal reaction. In rare severe cases insertion of a nasogastric tube for enteral hyperalimentation will be necessary.

Dermatitis: Because of the smaller volume of tissue in the supraclavicular fossae compared with the mid-chest, a higher dose per fraction will generally be delivered in this area unless special wedge compensator filters are used. Erythema, pruritus, dry and even moist desquamation can be seen in this area. Routine skin care should be applied.

Subacute and Chronic Reactions

Radiation pneumonitis: This is a clinical syndrome consisting of symptoms of cough, which may be non-productive early on but later productive of whitish or purulent sputum if a secondary infection ensues. Other symptoms include dyspnea, chest fullness and fever. Tachypnea and cyanosis can occur.

Radiation pneumonitis should be included in the differential diagnosis of any patient who has received radiation therapy to the thorax with symptoms. A chest radiograph will show infiltrates in the irradiated volume. Because contemporary radiation therapy involves the use of angled, shaped fields with sophisticated computer-assisted planning, the exact treatment volume should be discussed with the radiation therapist when this diagnosis is entertained. Often times, an infiltrate can be seen in part of the chest which one would not anticipate to have received a significant dose of radiation had the patient been treated with only opposing anterior and posterior portals. A CT scan may be helpful in finding radiation changes in relation to a treatment volume.

The timing of the appearance of the clinical radiation pneumonitis depends upon (1) the volume of lung parenchyma irradiated, (2) the fraction size, (3) the total dose, (4) the overall treatment time, (5) exposure to certain chemotherapeutic agents such as bleomycin, doxorubicin, actinomycin-D, BCNU and cyclophosphamide and (6) withdrawal of steroids. Generally, the characteristic radiographic findings are established by about 8 weeks after completion of a conventionally fractionated course of 4000 rad delivered over 4 weeks. For each 1000 rad increment above 4000 rad, Lipshitz and Southard predicted that radiation pneumonitis will appear 1 week earlier.

The treatment of radiation pneumonitis consists of supplemental oxygen if needed, prednisone in doses of 40-60 mg/day tapered slowly over a 4-6 week period and antibiotics as dictated by the presence of purulent sputum and/or positive cultures. The differential diagnosis includes primary infectious processes, lymphangitic spread of tumor, pulmonary toxicity from chemotherapy and locally recurrent tumor. Open thoracotomy with lung biopsy may be necessary to rule out pneumocystis, or other opportunistic infections.

Radiation fibrosis: This is a radiographic finding appearing 2-12 months following radiation therapy to the thorax and may be without associated symptoms. These changes are usually stable 9-12 months post-irradiation. The use of steroids has not been shown to prevent its development.

Some recent experimental work has shown that D-penicillamine can minimize the deposition of collagen in irradiated lung in rats and may have therapeutic implications in the future.

Esophageal stricture: This is a possible late complication seen when high doses are delivered to the mediastinum especially with the concomitant use of doxorubicin. This must be distinguished from recurrent tumor. Bougienage is the treatment of choice for benign stricture.

Pericarditis: When significant volumes of the heart are irradiated, a constrictive pericarditis may ensue months to years following treatment. If there is significant hemodynamic compromise, pericardial stripping can provide relief.

Transverse Myelitis: It is necessary to limit the dose to the spinal cord to 4500 rad to avoid this complication.

MESOTHELIOMA

OVERVIEW

Mesotheliomas may arise from the pleura, peritoneum, pericardium or tunica vaginalis. Pleural mesotheliomas, to be discussed below, account for approximately 70% of these tumors. The incidence in the general population is about 0.01%, increasing to 3% in populations exposed to asbestos. Asbestos exposure acts syngergistically with cigarette smoking in causing bronchogenic carcinoma but not mesotheliomas. Because of a 30-40 year lag period from the time of exposure to the development of mesothelioma, this disease may become increasingly important in the latter decades of this century.

PATHOLOGY & CLINICAL FEATURES

Mesothelioma occurs in a localized solitary form which is histologically benign and accounts for 25% of mesotheliomas. The remainder are of the diffuse malignant type. There are three histologic subtypes listed in Table 9.2.

Table 9.2
Malignant Mesothelioma - Subtypes

Histology	Frequency
Epithelial (tubopapillary)	50%
Fibrous (sarcoma)	25%
Biphasic, containing elements of both	25%

Special staining for mucin, hyaluornic acid, CEA and keratin as well as electron microscopic studies aid in the differential diagnosis. The clinical features of malignant mesothelioma often present as a recurrent pleural effusion, dyspnea and chest pain. A history of asbestos exposure has been reported in anywhere from 11 to 91% of patients in a variety of epidemiologic studies. The male to female ratio is 3:1.

STAGING

The Intergroup Mesothelioma Committee has proposed a clinical staging system for pleural mesothelioma. Its clinical utility has yet to be established since the results of treatment are generally poor regardless of stage. For Stage I patients with disease limited to the homolateral hemithorax, the median survival is 16 months. For Stage III patients with distant metastases, the median survival is reduced to 6 months.

WORK-UP

A histologic diagnosis is essential and most pathologists prefer open biopsies since it is very difficult to establish a diagnosis on the basis of pleural fluid cytology or a closed needle biopsy. Diffuse papillary mesothelioma may be difficult to differentiate from metastatic adenocarcinoma. Bronchoscopy is important to rule out an endobronchial lung cancer. CT scanning is helpful to define pleural-based masses and calcified pleural plaques. If a free pleural effusion is present, scanning should be done in the supine and lateral decubitus positions to adequately visualize the entire pleural surface.

TREATMENT and RESULTS

Treatment remains investigational. If a tumor is localized, surgery is occasionally curative. Various surgical procedures including radical pleurectomy and pleuropneumonectomy with or without diaphragmatic resection have their advocates. These formidable surgical resections carry up to a 20% perioperative mortality.

Although some long-term survivals have resulted to date, the median survival is little improved by radical radiation alone or in combination with surgery. The Intergroup Mesothelioma Committee is presently investigating multimodal management for malignant mesothelioma localized to one hemithorax. Surgery is followed by 4500 rad to the entire hemithorax, with a 1440 rad boost to residual pleural disease. The patients are then randomized to observation only or doxorubicin chemotherapy. Several authors have reported control of pleural effusion and palliation of chest pain with doses exceeding 4000 rads. Intracavitary colloidal gold-198 or P-32 have been utilized to control recurrent effusions.

THYMOMAS

OVERVIEW

Thymomas are rare intrathoracic tumors, although they are perhaps the most common tumors of the anterior mediastinum. These are discussed here because treatment techniques are similar to those used for bronchogenic carcinoma.

PATHOLOGY

Histologically it is difficult to distinguish benign thymomas from malignant thymomas. This distinction is best made on the basis of encapsulation and the presence or absence of invasion of adjacent tissues. This distinction is often more easily made grossly on the basis of pleural seeding or invasion of great vessels of nerves in the mediastinum. Histologic subtypes are lymphocytic, epithelial, lymphoepithelial (mixed) and spindle. Up to 66% are malignant.

CLINICAL FEATURES

Presenting symptoms are related to intrathoracic extension of tumor causing chest pain, superior vena caval obstruction or hoarseness from recurrent laryngeal nerve paralysis. Occasionally, a mediastinal mass will be noted in a routine chest radiograph. Tracheal invasion is an ominous sign. Rarely, there can be invasion of a major bronchi. There appears to be no predominance by sex.

There is a strong association between thymomas and myasthenia gravis with 10% of myasthenic patients having benign or malignant thymomas. Conversely, up to 50% of patients with malignant thymomas will have myasthenia gravis. Pure red cell aplasia occurs in 55% of thymoma patients.

STAGING

None in general use.

WORK-UP

This should proceed according to the work-up outline for lung cancer. Here, CT scan of the chest would be particularly helpful in defining a cystic component within tumors in the anterior mediastinum. Thoracotomy is also necessary to establish this diagnosis.

TREATMENT and RESULTS

For histologically and clnically benign thymomas total surgical excision is curative. For malignant tumors showing invasion, total excision is usually impossible and postoperative irradiation is mandatory as no long-term survivors were reported in a large series treated by surgery alone. Postoperative radiation therapy is recommended with minimum doses of 4500 rad to the entire mediastinum and supraclavicular nodal aarea following by 1000 to 1500 rad boost to areas of gross residual disease. Five year disease-free survival of 21% has been reported.

REFERENCES

1. Yarbro JW et al: Non-small cell carcinoma of the lung. Semin Oncol 10:1-126, 1983.
2. Perez C: Is postoperative irradiation indicated in carcinoma of the lung? I J Rad Onc Bio Phys8:2019-2022, 1982.
3. Cox JD, Komaki R and Byhardt RW: Is immediate chest radiotherapy obligatory for any or all patients with limited-stage non-small cell carcinoma of the lung? yes. Cancer Treatment Reports 67:327-331, 1983.
4. Byhardt RW and Cox JD: Is chest radiotherapy necessary in any or all patients with small cell carcinoma of the lung? yes. Cancer Treatment Reports 67:209-215, 1983.
5. Byhardt RW, Cox JD, Holoye PY et al: The role of consolidation irradiation in combined modality therapy of small cell carcinoma of the lung. I J Rad Onc Bio Phys 8:1271-1276, 1982.
6. Seydel HG, Creech RH, Mietlowski W et al: Radiation therapy in small cell lung cancer. Semin Oncol 5:288-298, 1978.
7. Salazar OM and Creech RH: "The state of the art" toward defining the role of radiation therapy in the management of small cell bronchogenic carcinoma. I J Rad Onc Bio Phys 6:1103-1117, 1980.
8. Katz H: The effect of rresection on local failure in irradiated non-oat cell carcinoma of the lung. I J Rad Onc Bio Phys (in press).
9. Chahinian AP, Pajak TF, Holland, JF et al: Diffuse malignant mesothelioma. Prospective evaluation of 69 patients. Ann Intern Med 96:746-755, 1982.
10. Chahinian AP, Bhardwaj S, Meyer RJ et al: Treatment of invasive or metastatic thymoma. Cancer 47:1752-1761, 1981.
11. Libshitz HL (ed), North LB: Lung. Diagnostic Roentgenology of Radiotherapy Change, pp 33-46, The Williams & Wilkins Co, Baltimore, MD, 1979.

Chapter 10

Gastrointestinal Cancer

ESOPHAGUS

OVERVIEW

Although palliation can be obtained in over 80% of patients with esophageal carcinoma, cure is uncommon because of the extent of disease at presentation. Radiation therapy can provide palliation with relatively little morbidity and may result in an occasional cure.

PATHOLOGY

Over 90% of esophageal carcinomas are squamous cell. Adenocarcinomas occur in the distal esophagus but frequently originate in the stomach. A columnar lined distal esophagus (Barrett's esophagus) is seen in up to 11% of patients with reflux esophagitis and adenocarcinoma can develop subsequently in 2 to 8% of such patients. Rare tumors of the esophagus include undifferentiated, oat cell and basal cell carcinomas, adenocanthoma, carcinosarcoma, mucoepidermoid and adenoid cystic adenocarcinoma, leiomyosarcoma, and malignant melanoma.

CLINICAL FEATURES

Esophageal cancer constitutes 1% of all cancer in North America and causes 2% of all deaths from cancer. It develops most frequently in the fifth and sixth decades of life, occuring three times more commonly in men than in women. Both hereditary and environmental factors have been implicated in its causation. Predisposing conditions include longstanding (> 25 years) achalasia, Plummer-Vinson syndrome, corrosive strictures and esophageal web.

For purposes of classification the esophagus is considered to consist of three principal regions:

1. Cervical esophagus - from the crico-pharyngeal sphincter to the thoracic inlet
2. Upper and mid-thoracic esophagus - from the thoracic inlet to 10 cm above the esophago-gastric junction
3. Lower thoracic esophagus - from 10 cm above the esophagogastric junction to the esophagogastric junction.

Dysphagia is the most common presenting symptom but does not occur until the circumference of the esophagus is narrowed one-half to one-third of normal. Weight loss is usually severe. Cough initiated by swallowing may indicate a tracheoesophageal fistula. Hoarseness may be dué to recurrent laryngeal nerve involvement in the mediastinum. Pain is a frequent complaint usually due to extraesophageal spread.

Local spread of the cancer is initially along the esophageal axis but less than 30% of tumors are confined to the esophagus at the time of presentation. Lymph node metastases develop early. Nearly 50% of patients with mid and distal esophageal tumors have involvement of the celiac nodes. Supraclavicular and mediastinal nodes are also often involved, depending on location of primary tumor. Distant metastases to lung or bone are common and correlate with the extent of the esophageal lesion.

STAGING:

TNM Staging for Esophageal Cancer

Primary Tumor (T)

T0	No demonstrable tumor
TIS	Carcinoma in situ
T1	Tumor involves 5 cm or less of esophageal length with no obstruction; no circumferential involvement no extraesophageal spread+
T2	Tumor involves more than 5 cm of esophagus and produces obstruction* with circumferential involvement of the esophagus but no extraesophageal spread
T3	Tumor with extraesophageal spread+

*Obstruction is defined by radiologic evidence of significant impediment to the passage of liquid contrast material past the tumor or endoscopic evidence of obstruction.
+Extraesophageal spread is defined by evidence of: (1) recurrent laryngeal, phrenic, or sympathetic nerve involvement; (2) fistula formation; (3) involvement of the tracheal or bronchial tree; (4) vena cava or azygous vein obstruction; (5) malignant effusion.

Regional Lymph Nodes (N)

Cervical esophagus (cervical and supraclavicular lymph nodes)

N0	No nodal involvement
N1	Unilateral involvement (movable)
N2	Bilateral involvement (movable)
N3	Fixed nodes

Thoracic esophagus (nodes in the thorax, not those of the cervical, supraclavicular or abdominal areas)

N0	No nodal involvement
N1	Nodal involvement

Distant Metastases

M0	No metastases
M1	Distant metastases. Cancer of thoracic esophagus with cervical, supraclavicular, or abdominal lymph node involvement is classified as M1

Stage Grouping for Esophageal Cancer

Stage I

T0, N0, M0	Tumor that involves less than 5 cm of eophagus without obstruction and no circumferential nor extraesophageal nor nodal involvement and no metastases.

Stage II

T1, N1, M0 T1, N2, M0 T2, N0, M0 T2, N1, M0 T2, N2, M0	Cervical esophagus: No extraesophageal involvement with moveable regional lymph nodes but no metastases, or a tumor, more than 5 cm in size without lymph node involvement. Thoracic esophagus: Any tumor which is greater than 5 cm in length or produces obstruction or involves the entire circumference of the esophagus without extraesophageal spread.

Stage III

Any M1	Any esophageal cancer with extraesophageal spread or distant metastases.
Any T3	Cervical esophagus: Fixed nodes (Any N3). Thoracic esophagus: Regional lymph node involvement (Any N1).

WORK-UP

Chest x-ray, esophagogram, esophagoscopy with cytology and biopsy, bone survey and bone scan, liver function tests and liver scan, CT scan of the thorax and abdomen are recommended.

The esophagogram, although useful in defining location, is not highly accurate in assessing the extent of the esophageal lesion. A CT scan of the thorax and upper abdomen may indicate extraesophageal spread and nodal involvement and is useful to the radiotherapist in treatment planning. Bronchoscopy is indicated with upper and mid-thoracic esophagus tumors since the possiblity of invasion of the trachea or bronchi often exists. Second primary lesions of the upper aerodigestive tract are not uncommon and should be ruled out by endoscopy. If surgery is being considered, mediastinoscopy may be needed to evaluate mediastinal nodal involvement. Celiac nodal biopsy is often performed at surgery prior to planned esophageal resections.

TREATMENT AND RESULTS

Radiation therapy is used in palliative and curative treatment of esophageal cancer either alone or in combination with surgery or chemotherapy. Radiation is often the primary treatment due to its palliative and occasionaly curative capability with relatively low morbidity.

Curative Treatment

Patients with Stage I, II and some with Stage III may be approached curatively. The significant mortality of surgical treatment (5-20%) limits its usefulness. Other than for localized adenocarcinoma of the distal esophagus, which may be best treated surgically, radiation therapy is usually recommended as the primary treatment.

Preoperative radiation has been used to shrink tumor and nodal metastases and increase resectability, but survival is not improved over either modality alone. Nakayama reported a five year survival of 37.5 % (3 of 8 patients at risk), but had a highly selected population that had to complete three separate surgical procedures.

Radiation alone (6000 rad in 6 weeks) results in local control in 30-50% of esophageal cancers. External beam irradiation is initially given to esophageal tumor plus a wide margin, and regional nodes to 5000 rad, followed by a boost to the to 6000 rad. Five-year survival with radiation alone is disappointingly low (5-10%).

Radiotherapy often fails because of tumor recurrence within the irradiated volume, but tumor dissemination is also frequent. A combination of radiation and concurrent chemotherapy (5-FU and Mitomycin) may offer promise in improving cure rates. No improved survival has yet been established, but local clearance rates of 60 to 80% have been obtained.

Postoperative radiation to decrease local recurrence is indicated when surgical margins are positive or gross disease remains. Prophylactic postoperative irradiation reportedly improves survival in patients undergoing a curative resection for thoracic esophageal carcinoma (5 year survival = 35%).

Palliation

Palliation alone should be the only goal in patients with: (1) Distant metastses. (2) Primary lesions greater than 10 cm. (3) Suspected perforation or tracheoesophageal fistula.

Radiation can relieve dysphagia in 60-80% of patients for an average duration of about six months. Typically, 4000-5000 rad are given in four to five weeks. Dysphagia may improve within the first two weeks of treatment. Radiation is not given to patients with tracheoesophageal fistula since benefit is rarely obtained. Patients with tracheal invasion but no fistula may be treated effectively with radiation.

Dilatation, intraluminal bypass devices, and various surgical procedures may be used to bypass esophageal obstruction when radiation does not suffice. If necessary, dilatation can be performed in patients undergoing radiotherapy. Long-term gastrostomy should be avoided since esophageal stenosis may result from lack of physiologic peristalsis and dilatation. Additionally, in the presence of total obstruction, patients cannot handle secretions and aspiration is common. Parentereal nutrition is very important in patients with obstruction.

Chemotherapy presently shows little usefulness in the treatment of disseminated esophageal carcinoma.

MORBIDITY

Acute

Esophagitis: Most patients will experience a transient esophagitis around the third week of treatment. Conservative management with Oxaine-M or viscous xylocaine and analgesics usually will suffice in reducing discomfort. Moniliasis may occur and should be vigorously treated.

Tracheal-esophageal fistula: Rapid tumor reduction by radiation may result in fistula formation when there is initial evidence of tracheal invasion. Some radiotherapists will, therefore, decrease the daily dose to minimize this complication. Fistula formation has been reported to occur in 5-18% of irradiated patients. Recurrent tumor may also result in a fistula.

Chronic

Esophageal ulceration and stricture: These late-occuring side effects four to six months post radiation are seen in less than 5% of patients treated to 6300 rad. When doses exceed 6650 rad, as many as 50% of patients may have these complications.

Pneumonitis: Careful treatment planning which minimizes radiation dose to the lung results in a low incidence of pneumonitis (less than 10%). When bleomycin is given with radiation, pulmonary toxicity may be prohibitive depending on the volume of lung irradiated.

Others: Esophageal perforation and mediastinitis, myelitis, pericarditis (rare).

STOMACH

OVERVIEW

The incidence of stomach cancer in the United States has decreased from 30/100,000 in 1930 to 8/100,000 in 1980. Migrant populations from high risk countries (e.g. Japan, 78/100,000) to the U.S. show a significant decrease in disease occurrrence suggesting an environmental or dietary etiology.

Surgery remains the primary treatment of gastric malignancies. High doses of radiation are precluded due to the limited tolerance of the stomach and surrounding upper abdominal structures to radiation. Techniques such as intraoperative radiation are under investigation in an attempt to diminish problems with normal tissue irradiation. Radiation therapy may be useful in improving local control and offering palliation. Advanced gastric cancers, unlike other gastrointestinal malignancies have a high response rate to combination chemotherapy (40-60%).

PATHOLOGY

Adenocarcinoma comprises the vast majority of gastric malignancies (95%) while lymphomas are rare (less than 5%). Others include leiomyosarcomas, adenoacanthomas, squamous cell carcinomas and carcinoid tumors.

Most gastric cancers occur in the antrum or lower one-third of the stomach. The lesser curvature gives rise to cancers more frequently than the greater curvature. Multicentric cancers are found histologically in over 20% of patients with gastric carcinoma.

Gastric cancers can be divided in four categroies on the basis of gross pathologic features (See Table 10.1). Microscopic features such as the degree of differentiation often correlate with gross pathology.

Table 10.1
Categories of Gastric Carcinoma.

Type	% Occurrence	Gross Features	Usual Degree of Differentiation
Ulcerative	> 75%	Ulcer, invasive mass	Poor
Polypoid	10%	Large mass little invasion	Well
Scirrhous	10%	Thick rigid wall	Poor (anaplastic)
Superficial	< 5%	Sheet like tumor replacing normal mucosa	Moderate

CLINICAL FEATURES

Pain, weight loss and vomiting are the most common symptoms of gastric malignancy.

Adenocarcinoma: Although ulcerative gastric cancer is common, it rarely arises from pre-existing benign gastric ulcers. Multiple paths of spread exist. Most tumors are advanced, 80% with lymph node involvement, 40% peritoneal involvement and 33% with hepatic metastases at diagnosis.

Lymphoma: Gastric lymphomas are usually solitary, diffuse histiocytic tumors and average about 6-7 cm. in greatest dimension at diagnosis. Regional nodes are involved in about 40% of patients.

STAGING

None in common usage.

WORK-UP

1. History and physical exam: Attention to potential sites of spread that may be biopsied

-supraclavicular nodes, liver. Rectal exam may reveal a Blumer's shelf due to pelvic peritoneal spread.

2. Radiologic studies: UGI with double contrast, chest x-ray, liver scan.
3. Endoscopy with biopsy and cytology.
4. Laboratory studies: CBC, SMA-12.
5. Optional: CT abdomen to evaluate for peritoneal deposits, liver extention etc.
6. Diagnostic/therapeutic laparotomy and resection.

TREATMENT AND RESULTS

Adenocarcinoma: The primary treatment is surgical with a some form of subtotal gastrectomy the procedure of choice, though the approach must be individualized based on the extent of tumor. Five-year survival is only 10%; however, it is 60% in patients without nodal involvement. Postoperative adjuvant radiotherapy may have a role in reducing local failure and improving survival in patients with lymph node involvement or penetration of the tumor through the gastric wall. Several protocols exist to study the effectiveness of adjuvant chemotherapy plus or minus radiotherapy. Intraoperative radiotherapy has been curative in some patients with incompletely excised tumors. Patients with unresectable tumors have a median survival of one year when treated with radiation and 5-FU compared to six months with radiation alone.

Effective combination chemotherapy exists for advanced gastric cancer. Use of 5-FU, doxorubicin and mitomycin (FAM) has resulted in objective response rates of 40-60%. Significant responses can be seen even with large intra-abdominal disease. The treatment is well tolerated and responders have an improved performance status.

Lymphomas: Radiation alone can be curative even with advanced tumors but because of the possibility of perforation during treatment and the additional information gained by laparotomy, surgery (partial gastrectomy) is indicated in most patients. Surgery is curative in 80-90% of early cancers with only submucosal invasion, but when the gastric wall has been penetrated or regional lymph nodes involved, the survival drops to 25-35%. Postoperative radiotherapy decreases local recurrence in such locally invasive cases. Chemotherapy may also be of value, particularly in advanced presentations.

MORBIDITY

Acute

Nausea and vomiting frequently accompany gastric radiation and may be controlled with Compazine.

Chronic

Gastric ulcers - Doses of over 5000 rad may produce gastric ulcers two or more months following completion of radiation. A medical regimen of antacids and cimetidine usually allows healing.

Nephritis can occur if radiotherapy techniques do not exclude at least two-thirds of one kidney.

PANCREAS

OVERVIEW

Carcinoma of the pancreas is a debilitating and usually fatal disease. Recent aggressive approaches in radiation therapy for locally advanced disease have improved median survival to about one year. Five-year survival remains less than 5%.

PATHOLOGY

Eighty-five percent of pancreatic carcinomas are adenocarcinomas with duct cell adenocarcinoma the most frequent type. Other histologic types include giant cell, acinar cell, adenosquamous and cystadenocarcinoma. Fibrosis and pancreatitis almost always accompany pancreatic cancer and may comprise two-thirds of gross pancreatic mass seen at surgery. Multifocal carcinoma remote from the gross disease may be present in 25% of patients.

Tumors of the endocrine pancreas may be of islet cell or interacinar cell origin. They are part of the APUD system and give rise to several distinct syndromes.

CLINICAL FEATURES

Weight loss is seen in over 90% of patients with pancreatic cancer regardless of its location in the pancreas. The pancreatic head is involved in two-thirds of patients. Most patients present with progressive jaundice and pain. The one-third of tumors located in the body or tail of the pancreas are usually quite large before symptoms develop and diagnosis is made. Nodal involvement is present in 80-90% of patients.

Rarely, acinar cell carcinomas may be assciated with elevated serum and tumor lipase levels, panniculitis, essinophelia, arthralgias and arthritis.

Cystadenocarcinoma, which comprises about 1% of pancreatic cancer, has a relatively good prognosis. It usually arises in the tail of the pancreas and presents as a large mucinous-containing abdominal mass. Surgical resection results in 30-60% long-term survival.

STAGING

None in common usage.

WORK-UP

History and physical exam should be performed with attention to areas of potential spread that may be biopsied, e.g. supraclavicular nodes, liver. Abdominal ultrasound, pancreatic function tests and ERCP provide the diagnosis with 90% accurarcy. CT scan is useful in defining the extent of the disease and detecting liver involvement. Chest x-ray and routine lab needed prior to surgery.

TREATMENT AND RESULTS

Surgery

Carcinomas of the pancreas which are localized with no invasion of the liver, superior mesenteric artery or inferior vena cava have been treated with radical pancreaticoduodenectomy (Whipple's procedure) with poor results. Morbidity and mortality from this procedure are high. Median survival is less than one year and five-year survival is less than 10%.

Surgery plays an important role in unresectable pancreatic cancers which will be treated with radiotherapy plus or minus chemotherapy. Useful surgical procedures include:

1. Pancreatic biopsy to establish diagnosis.
2. Regional nodal biopsy and biopsy of suspicious areas to identify disease extent.
3. If interstitial radioactive iodine implant is planned, the surgeons can expose the tumor for the radiotherapist. The tumor is then implanted and bypass procedures can be performed.
4. Placement of metallic clips at the margins of disease in all three dimensions outlines the tumor volume for external beam radiotherapy treatment planning.
5. Palliative bypass procedures, usually cholecystojejunostomy and gastrojejunostomy. Anastomosis should be placed out of the intended radiation field, if possible. Omentum placed under the stomach may move the stomach away from the pancreas and out of the high dose target volume, thus decreasing problems associated with gastric radiation.

Radiotherapy

High dose external beam radiotherapy (greater than 6000 rad) has resulted in survival comparable to Whipple's procedure (median 10-12 months, 5-year less than 10%). Local control is less than 50%. Pain palliation is obtained in the majority of patients. Morbidity of radiation, including gastritis and bleeding, is seen in less than 10% of patients when treatment planning techniques are used to exclude most of the stomach and bowel from the high dose volume.

Because of poor local control with external beam radiation alone, interstitial radiation with an I-125 implant has been used initially followed by 4000-5000 rad in 5 weeks to the tumor and regional nodes with external beam radiation. Doses of 12,000-16,000 rad are typically delivered to the implanted tumor volume during the decay of iodine-125 with about 90% of that dose given during the first 6 months following the implant. Thus far, although local control may be improved by implant, survival is similar to external beam radiation alone. Distant metastases are present in about 80% of patients who fail treatment. Complications of implant may include pancreatic fistula formation in up to 20% of patients. Administration of 5-FU concurrently with radiation appears to increase median survival over radiation alone.

Combination chemotherapy, particular regimens containing 5-FU and mitomycin have some effectiveness in the the treatment of advanced disseminated disease. Patients with prior abdominal irradiation should probably start at a decreased chemotherapeutic dosage to avoid hematologic problems.

MORBIDITY

Combined modality treatment of pancreatic cancer requires dilligent patient support. Significant psychosocial problems usually exist in this debilitating disease. Following I-125 implant, post-surgical complications of wound dehiscence and infection, bowel obstruction and pulmonary embolism may occur. Pancreatic pseudocyst formation is uncommon following an implant. Most patients resume eating within one week post-surgery. External beam treatment is fairly well tolerated with over 80% of patients completing a full course of radiation. Patients lose an average of 7 lbs. during treatment. The majority have exocrine pancreas insufficiency which responds moderately to enzyme supplements. Less than 10% suffer from radiation induced gastritis or bleeding. No renal, hepatic or hematologic toxicity is reported following radiation with careful treatment planning. A high rate of death from intercurrent disease is a problem in long-term survivors (> 1 year).

COLORECTAL

OVERVIEW

Colorectal carcinoma is second only to lung cancer as the leading cause of cancer deaths in the United States. Surgery is the primary treatment but radiotherapy is useful: (1) Preoperatively to make unresectable lesions resectable. (2) Pre and postoperatively to decrease local recurrence and improve surival. (3) Alone to provide palliation and occasional cure of advanced or inoperable disease.

PATHOLOGY

Adenocarcinomas comprise most colorectal cancers. Carcinoid tumors and lymphomas are occasionally found. Cloacogenic tumors originate in the anal region below the pectinate line. Squamous cell carcinomas of the anus occur infrequently.

CLINICAL FEATURES

Colorectal cancer occurs most frequently in patients over 60 years of age. The male to female ratio is about equal. Fifty percent of colorectal cancers occur in the rectum and 20% in the sigmoid.

Colorectal polyps may give rise to carcinoma. Adenomatous polyps occur frequently but have relatively low invasive potential (< 5%). About one in ten colorectal polyps is a villous adenoma. These have nearly ten times the malignant potential of adenomatous polyps. Nearly all patients with familial polyposis develop carcinoma. Ulcerative colitis is associated with increased risk of colorectal cancer. Diets low in fiber and high in fat have been implicated as possible etiologic factors in the development of colorectal cancer.

The most frequent presenting symptoms depend on the location of tumor: rectal lesions - hematochezia, left colon - obstruction, right colon - anemia and right-lower quadrant pain.

Unlike esophageal carcinoma, longitudinal spread is usually not extensive, averaging only 1-2 cm from the gross disease. Over 25% of colon cancers have extended through the bowel wall. Cancers of the rectosigmoid have spread through the wall in 50-70% and metastasized to lymph nodes in 50-60%.

STAGE

Duke's (Astler-Collier Modification)

- A: Lymph nodes negative. Limited to mucosa.
- B1: Extension through mucosa but still within bowel wall; nodes negative.
- B2: Extension through entire bowel wall; nodes negative.
- C1: Lesion limited to bowel wall; nodes positive.
- C2: Extension through entire bowel wall; nodes positive.
- D: Distant metastases.

WORK-UP

Work-up should include history and physical with digital rectal examination, stool sample for occult blood, barium enema with air contrast, proctosigmoidoscopy, CEA, liver function tests. Liver scan, bone scan, colonoscopy, and IVP (if indicated). A CT scan of the pelvis should be done for treatment planning purposes in patients receiving radiotherapy.

TREATMENT AND RESULTS

COLON

Cancer of the ascending, transverse and descending colon is treated surgically with partial colectomy. The role of adjuvant radiotherapy and chemotherapy has not been clearly defined.

RECTOSIGMOID

Cancer of the rectosigmoid is also managed surgically with a low-anterior resection or, for low rectal lesions, with an abdominoperineal resection. Pelvic recurrence is less than 10% and five-year survival over 90% for patients with Duke's A or B1 malignancies. Unfortunately, the majority of tumors are more advanced and pelvic recurrence increases to 40-50% for lesions through the bowel wall (B2) and up to 70% when nodes are also involved (C2). Five-year survival for Duke's B2 and C rectosigmoid carcinomas is only 20-35% following surgery alone. Adjuvant 5-FU is used in combination with postoperative radiation to decrease local recurrence and improve survival.

Postoperative radiation of 4500-5000 rad to the whole pelvis reduces local failure in Duke's B2 and C malignancies to less than 10%. Survival of patients with such lesions is probably also improved, with some studies showing an overall 5-year survival of over 50% for patients with Duke's B2 and C disease treated with postoperative radiation. Postoperative radiation has the advantage of accurate surgical staging and may spare irradiation of patients with early disease (Duke's A and B1) and advanced disease (liver metastases). Residual masses or areas at risk for tumor recurrence should be marked with metalic clips at the time of surgical resection for subsequent radiotherapy treatment planning.

Preoperative radiation (4000-5000 rad) has also been shown to decrease pelvic recurrence rate and may improve survival. Preoperative radiation may also decrease the chance of intraoperative tumor dissemination.

Excellent local control rates (greater than 90%) and 5-year surival (66%) have been obtained for patients with Dukes B2 and C disease using the "sandwich technique" of combining surgery and radiation. With this technique preoperative radiation of 500 rad is given one day prior to surgery and postoperative radiation of 4500-5000 rad is started 3-6 weeks following surgery.

About one-half of patients with unresectable lesions who receive 4500-5000 rad will have sufficient decrease in the tumor extent to undergo resection within 4-6 weeks following radiation. Overall 5-year survival is up to 25-35% with this approach.

Primary Radiation

For selected low-lying rectal adenocarcinomas, contact radiotherapy alone may be curative. These malignancies must be well differentiated carcinomas without invasion of the bowel wall. Additionally, they must be less than 5 cm in greatest dimension and no further than 12 cm (though 7 cm or less is better) from the anal verge. Approximately 10,000-15,000 rad are delivered in 4 weekly doses on a 50 kv superficial x-ray unit. Local control is over 90% in this selected group.

Primary radiotherapy and chemotherapy (5-FU and mitomycin) have been successfully used in the treatment of cloacogenic carcinomas and squamous cell carcinomas of the anus.

Palliation

Surgical resection and/or diversion, when possible, are the most effective means of palliating obstructive symptoms. Radiation is only moderately effective in palliation. High radiation doses are usually required (> 5000 rad). Pain is decreased in 80% of patients irradiated, although only 20% report complete relief. Bleeding may be controlled in over 70%. Recurrent rectal cancers are controlled locally in about 15% of patients treated with radiation with a median survival of under two years. Patients with mobile, less advanced pelvic recurrences may do much better, particularly when surgical resection is possible.

MORBIDITY

Acute Reactions

Doses of 4000-5000 rad to the pelvis are usually well tolerated. Diarrhea frequently occurs during radiation. Dietary modifications to exclude fiber may be useful. Lomotil usually controls the diarrhea. Dysuria may also occur and can be controlled with analgesics or Pyridium. If the radiation field includes the perineum (as after A-P resections), there may be a brisk perineal skin reaction which heals with conservative management.

Chronic

Radiation proctitis, ulceration and bleeding are rarely seen with doses under 5500-6000 rad. Onset is usually 6-12 months following radiation. Conservative management with Lomotil, steroids, and steroid enemas often suffice to allow healing, but a colostomy may be required if symptoms persist or progress.

Radiation specific small bowel damage or adhesions leading to obstruction or perforation is seen in less than 5% of patients receiving 5000 rad pelvic irradiation. This risk is increased in patients with prior surgery or pelvic infection and large radiation doses or volumes.

MORBIDITY OF IRRADIATION OF SPECIFIC GI SITES

Stomach: Gastric irradiation occurs in the treatment of upper abdominal malignancies (e.g. cancers of stomach or pancreas or metastasic or lymphomatous involvement of para-aortic lymph nodes). Low doses of gastric irradiation (1500 to 2000 rad) result in decreased acid and pepsin secretion about one month following radiation and were once used to manage peptic ulcers when other measures failed. The reduction in acidity was not permanent and frequent re-irradiation resulted in significant damage to the stomach, occasionally with ulceration and perforation. When the stomach is included in para-aortic nodal irradiation, nausea may ensue after several treatments but is usually quite mild. Chronic changes post-gastric irradiation, usually atrophy and ulceration, may occur several months to one year after radiation doses of 4500 rad or more.

Liver: The relatively low liver tolerance to radiation presents a limitation to irradiation of the upper abdomen. Radiation damage to the endothelial cells results in centriloblular necrosis at relatively low doses. When the whole liver is irradiated at 200 rad daily , radiation hepatitis may be occasionally (less than 5%) observed at doses as low as 2500 rad. Patients receiving whole liver irradiation to 4000 rad may have up to a 50% risk of developing hepatitis. When treating the upper abdomen in ovarian cancer with the moving strip technique (See Chapter 12), the liver dose is limited to 2250 rad. Partial liver radiation rarely results in clinical radiation hepatitis if more than 1/3 of the liver is excluded.

Clinically in acute radiation hepatitis, hepatomegaly is often present along with ascites and elevated liver enzymes. This may occur 2-6 weeks following radiation. A liver scan usually shows a sharply demarcated area of decreased uptake corresponding to the radiation field. Alkaline phosphatase is moderately elevated and slight elevations in SGOT, SGPT and bilirubin may also be seen. Chronic radiation hepatitis occurs 4-6 months or more post-radiation and manifests as cirrhosis with centrilobular scarring resulting in portal hypertension and closely resembles the Budd-Chiari syndrome. Management is as with non-radiation hepatitis.

REFERENCES

1. Beatty JD et al: Carcinoma of the esophagus. Cancer 43:2254-2267, 1979.
2. Heit HA et al: Palliative dilation for dysphagia in esophageal carcinoma. Ann Int Med 89:629-631, 1978.
3. Kasai M et al: Follow-up results after resection of thoracic esophageal carcinoma. World J Surg 2:543-551, 1978.
4. Nakayama K: Surgical treatment combined with pre-opertive concentrated radiation for esophageal carcinoma. JAMA 227:178, 1974.
5. Pearson J.: Present status and future potential of radiotherapy in the management of esophageal carcinoma. Cancer 50:2590-2596, 1982.
6. Wara WM, Mauch PM, Thomas AN, Philips TL: Palliation for carcinoma of the esophagus. Radiology 121:717-721, 1976.
7. Carter SK, Comis RL: Gastric cancer: Current status of treatment. J Nat Cancer Inst 58:567-578, 1977.
8. Douglas HD: Potentially curable cancer of the stomach. Cancer 50:2582-2589, 1982.
9. Schein P et al: Current management of advanced and locally unresectable gastric carcinoma. Cancer 50:2590-2596, 1982.

10. Dobelbower RR: The radiotherapy of pancreatic cancer. _Semin Oncol_ 6:378, 1979.
11. Gunderson LL, Sosin H: Areas of failure found at reoperation for adenocarcinoma of the rectum. _Cancer_ 34:1278-1292, 1974.
12. Kligerman M: Radiotherapy and rectal cancer. _Cancer_ 39:896-900, 1977.
13. Mohiuddin M et al: Adjuvant radiotherapy with selective sandwich technique in the treatment of rectal cancer. _Dis Colon Rectum_ 24:76-79, 1981.
14. Papillion J: Resectable rectal cancer. Treatment by curative endocavitary irradiation. _JAMA_ 23:1385-1387, 1975.
15. Sischy B: The place of radiotherapy in the management of rectal adenocarcinoma. _Cancer_ 50:2631-2637, 1982.

Chapter 11

Genitourinary Cancer

RENAL CARCINOMA (Adult)

OVERVIEW

Adult kidney malignancies may arise from the renal parenchyma or renal pelvis. Primary treatment is surgical, although radiation and chemotherapy (including hormonal management) may also be used. Local recurrence alone is not a significant pattern of failure (less than 20%). Follow-up must be long because of the propensity for late metastases and the often unpredictable nature of this malignancy.

PATHOLOGY

Approximately 80% arise in the renal parenchyma as adenocarcinoma (hypernephroma). Twenty percent arise in the renal pelvis; the majority of these are transitional cell carcinomas, although squamous cell carcinomas are also found. Tumor grade is a major factor in determining prognosis, since high grade lesions have a greater incidence of invasion and metastasis than low grade.

CLINICAL FEATURES

Most renal cancers occur in the 50-60 age group. There is a 2:1 male predominance. Typical presenting symptom is hematuria. Associated flank pain is seen in about half the patients. An abdominal flank mass may also be present. Unusual features include fever (16%) and polycythemia (3%). Only 9% of patients present with the classic triad of gross hematuria, abdominal mass and pain.

Hypernephromas have spread through the renal capsule in nearly half of all patients at presentation. Distant metastases are seen at presentation in about one-third of patients. Bilateral cancers occur in 18% of patients. About 1% of patients will have spontaneous regression of their malignancy.

Transitional cell cancer of the renal pelvis is associated with a high risk of multiple carcinomas in the renal pelvis and ureter and may extend directly into the ureter and bladder.

STAGING

Renal adenocarcinoma. A TNM classification also exists.

Stage I: Tumor confined to the kidney.
Stage II: Tumor locally invasive but confined to Gerota's fascia.
Stage III: Regional invasion.
- A - Invasion of renal vein or vena cava or both.
- B - Metastases to regional lymph nodes.
- C - Combination of A and B.

Stage IV:
- A - Invasion of surrounding organs (other than adrenal glands).
- B - Distant metastases.

WORK-UP

The following are recommended for initial work-up:

History and physical exam (attention to flank mass, lower extremity edema). Urinalysis and urine cytology, IVP, chest x-ray, SMA-12 (liver chemistries and serum calcium), bone scan. CBC to evaluate for polycythemia or anemia. CT examination may differentiate cysts from solid tumor. Cysts can be aspirated percutaneously for cytologic exam if suspicious. An arteriogram is highly accurate in diagnosis of hypernephromas due to tumor neovascularity.

TREATMENT AND RESULTS

HYPERNEPHROMA

Definitive Treatment

Radical nephrectomy is the preferred treatment for all localized or locally advanced malignancies. Involvement of the renal vein or vena cava does not preclude surgery. Renal vein involvement may not be associated with a worse prognosis despite its importance in the present staging system. Hypernephroma may recur or metastasize many years after initial diagnosis and survival following treatment continues to diminish even past five years (See Table 11.1). Bilateral renal carcinoma is treated with nephrectomy for the larger tumor and partial nephrectomy for the smaller tumor.

Radiation has limited usefulness in the treatment of stage II and III hyprenephroma. Preoperative radiation of 4500 rad improves resectability in patients with advanced unresectable disease but has not been shown conclusively to affect survival. Postoperative radiation of 4500-5000 rad may improve local control and possibly survival of patients with invasion of the perinephric fat, lymphatics or vessels. Primary radiation is rarely used except in nonresectable tumors and is palliative.

Palliation

Patients with metastatic disease may rarely benefit from palliative nephrectomy and hormonal therapy (progesterone, testosterone). Isolated metastases to bone or lung may be treated with radiation or surgery. Despite claims that hypernephromas are radioresistant, effective palliation can be obtained by irradiating recurrent or metastatic sites.

Table 11.1
Survival for Hypernephroma

Stage	5-Year	10-Year
I & II	40-65%	25-45%
III	20-25%	15%
IV	5%	0%

RENAL PELVIC CARCINOMAS

Nephroureterectomy is the treatment of choice for cancers of the renal pelvis. There is no proven role for postoperative radiation. Overall 5-year survival is 30-40% for transitional cell carcinomas. Papillary transitional carcinomas without muscle wall invasion have a better 5-year survival (52%) than with invasion (17%). Squamous cell carcinomas have a very poor prognosis, with only rare 5-year survivors.

MORBIDITY

Acute

Since a large amount of bowel is irradiation with pre or postoperative irradiation of renal tumors, patients may experience nausea, vomiting and diarrhea.

Chronic (The late effects of kidney irradiation)

Radiation Nephritis: Pathophysiologically, radiation damage to renal microvasculature results in glomerular dysfunction at relatively low radiation doses (400 rad). Higher doses may produce structural and functional changes in all renal structures.

Clinically, development of radiation nephritis is a function of radiation dose and kidney volume irradiated. It may occur if both kidneys are irradiated to doses of 2300 rad in 5 weeks. One-third to one-half of a kidney may receive doses of 4000 rad or more without development of nephritis. Proteinuria, hypertension, edema, anemia and cardiomegaly may occur several months after radiation. Irradiation of only one kidney to high doses can produce malignant hypertension which will resolve after nephrectomy.

Careful medical management is necessary for patients with azotemia due to nephritis as with other causes of renal failure. Decreased dietary protein and salt restriction are generally useful. Corticosteroids are contraindicated. A BUN of greater than 100 and massive edema are associated with a worse prognosis.

BLADDER

OVERVIEW

Bladder cancer is the most frequent urinary tract malignancy and accounts for 3% of all cancer deaths in the United States. A combined approach of surgery and radiation is used in all but the earliest of bladder tumors and is generally felt to be superior to either treatment used alone.

PATHOLOGY

Approximately 90% of bladder tumors are transitional cell and about 10% are squamous cell, with adenocarcinoma occurring rarely. Transitional cell cancers usually appear in the posterior and lateral bladder walls but the trigone and dome are also occasionally involved. The most important prognosticator is depth of invasion into the bladder wall. Extension through the bladder wall increases pelvic lymph node involvement from less than 20% to over 50%. Histologic grade is also a significant prognostic factor. Low grade B1 cancers are associated with lymph node involvement in less than 25% compared to 40-50% with high grade B1 cancers. Tumors that have lost their ABO (H) antigen expression, but are of low histologic grade, non-invasive or superficially invasive, have a greater liklihood of subsequent recurrence and dissemination than similar tumors that have not loss this antigenic expression.

CLINICAL FEATURES

Bladder cancer is a disease of the 50-70 year age group with a 2.3:1 male predominance. Tobacco use, aniline dye and chemical exposure, as well as chronic bladder irritants (including cytoxan), are associated with bladder cancer. Patients with bilharzial affected bladders have an increased incidence of squamous cell carcinomas of the bladder. Congenital bladder extrophy is associated with adenocarcinoma.

Gross hematuria is the most frequent presenting symptom. Dysuria, frequency and urgency are present in 30-50% of patients.

STAGING

Two staging systems are in use; the TNM and Jewett-Marshall Classification are compared below.

Jewett-Marshall Staging	Depth of Invasion	TNM Classification: Clinical	TNM Classification: Pathological
0	No tumor in specimen	T0	P0
	Carcinoma in situ	TIS	PIS
	Papillary tumor without invasion		
A	Invasion lamina propria	T1	P1
B1	Superficial muscle invasion	T2	P2
B2	Deep muscle invasion	T3A	P3
C	Invasion of perivesical fat	T3B	
D1	Invasion of contiguous viscera	T4A	P4
	Pelvic nodes	N1-3	
D2	Distant mets	M1	
	Nodes above the bifurcation	N4	

WORK-UP

The work-up should include the history and physical exam along with routine studies including chest x-ray, urinalysis, IVP, cystoscopy, exam under anesthesia and biopsy, CBC & SMA 12, bone and liver scans. Also, CT scanning, transurethral ultrasound, ABO(H) antigen testing and flow cytometry show potential in aiding the evaluation of new or recurrent bladder cancers.

TREATMENT AND RESULTS

Therapy of bladder cancer is dependent on a number of factors besides tumor stage. The grade and location of the tumor determine the extent of regional treatment necessary. The general health of the patient and prior therapies may limit the ability of the patient to tolerate some procedures (See Table 11.2).

Low grade superficial bladder cancer (O,A) may be managed with transurethral resection, intravesical installation of thiotepa and other chemotherapy or BCG. Multiple recurrences are often more deeply invasive and may require cystectomy or radiation therapy. Five-year survival is 60-70%. High grade superficial tumors (O,A) are relatively uncommon. They tend to recur locally and are often treated with cystectomy or radiation.

Low grade B1 lesions may be treated with segmental resection if solitary and located on the dome or on the lateral walls and if a 3 cm margin of resection can be obtained. Radioactive implants can be used instead of resection if the lesion is accessible with similarly good results.

High grade B1 lesions have a significant incidence of regional nodal metastases and are generally treated with combined modality therapy as are Stage B2 and C lesions. Preoperative radiation of various doses (2000 rad in one week to 5000 rad in 5 weeks) have been used and may result in an increased 5-year survival (50%) over radiation or cystectomy alone (20-25%). At Jefferson Hospital, with 500 rad pre-op and 4500 rad postoperative radiation, a 5-year survival of 55-65% of patients treated for high grade B1, B2 or C lesions is reported.

Curative use of radiation therapy alone for inoperable or unresectable patients requires high doses of 6500-7000 rad in 7-8 weeks to be delivered to the tumor. Although about 20-30% of patients treated with radiation alone will be 5-year survivors, selected patients with good bladder function who wish to preserve their bladders may fare better. Such patients include those with T2 and T3 tumors without ureteral obstruction and with "complete" resection at TURB. Salvage cystectomy may be possible in up to 50% of patients who fail with high dose radiation.

Table 11.2
Summary of commonly used Treatment Regimens and Survival in Bladder Cancer

STAGE	GRADE	LOCATION	TREATMENT	5-YR SURVIVAL
O,A	Low	Local	Transurethral resection or intravesicle installation of chemo or BCG	60-70%
O,A	High	Multiple	Cystectomy or radiation to bladder only	60%
B1	Low	Dome Lateral wall	Segmental resection	50%
B1	High	Any	Pre or post-op radiation and cystectomy	40-65%
B2,C	Any	Any	Pre or post-op radiation and cystectomy	40-65%

MORBIDITY

Acute

Acute cystitis occurs after 3000-4000 rad in the majority of patients. Symptoms of bladder irritation, dysuria, frequency and urgency are seen. Infection may accompany cystitis and a urine culture should be obtained. Pyridium 100-200 mg b.i.d. or Urispas 100 mg q.i.d. usually relieves discomfort. Daily radiation may have to be diminished or temporarily stopped if cystitis is not responsive to these medications. Acute cystitis subsides within 2 weeks after completion of radiation.

Late

Chronic cystitis occurs 6 months after high dose radiation. Less than 5% of patients treated to 5000 rad or less will develop chronic problems due to contracted bladder. As dose increases to 6500-7000 rad, 15% of patients will experience considerable contraction or hemorrhagic cystitis.

The risk of developing chronic cystitis is diminished if radiation is not administered until 4-6 weeks following TUR. Bladder infections should be controlled, and mechanical instrumentation and catheterization avoided or minimized during radiation.

PROSTATE

OVERVIEW

Cancer of the prostate is the most common cancer in men over 50 years of age (excluding skin). When disease is localized, surgery or radiotherapy offer good chances for cure. Lymph node involvement or elevated acid phosphatase are associated with a poorer prognosis. Hormonal manipulation is useful in palliative therapy. Follow-up must be long, since late recurrence and metastases are frequent.

PATHOLOGY

Adult prostatic cancers are almost exclusively adenocarcinomas. Two histologic grading systems are used. The system of Mostofi looks at cellular detail and histologic pattern to define 3 grades: (1) well differentiated, (2) moderately differentiated, and (3) poorly differentiated or anaplastic. Gleason's system is based on major and minor histologic patterns observed. Numbers from 1 to 5 (well differentiated to poorly differentiated) are assigned to both major and minor patterns. The sum of the two numbers (Gleason score) ranges from 2 to 10 and correlates with the survival and incidence of nodal involvement. Additionally, one can add a number (from 1 to 5) corresponding to clinical stage to the Gleason score to obtain a stage-histologic pattern category (Gleason category) which correlates even better with prognosis.

CLINICAL FEATURES

Stage A lesions (10%) are usually found incidentally. These patients frequently present with symptoms of outlet obstruction with a normal rectal examination, but disease is found on review of pathologic specimen from transurethral resection of the prostate. Stage A2 lesions are usually poorly differentiated adenocarcinomas and have a 25% incidence of pelvic lymph node involvement.

Patients with Stage B lesions (5-10%) may or may not have outlet obstruction symptoms, and are found to have prostatic abnormality confined to the prostate gland.

The majority of patients present with advanced disease (Stage C, 45% or Stage D, 40%). Advanced lesions occasionally cause ureteral obstruction or painful bone metastases.

Approximately 85% of prostatic cancer affects the posterior lobes; 15% are located anteriorly and cannot be easily palpated unless advanced.

Regional nodal involvement correlates with the size of the lesion and degree of differentiation. Less than 10% of Stage A1 lesions have lymph node involvement compared to an average of 20% for Stage B and 65% for Stage C. Gleason's scores of 2-5 are associated with 14% lymph node involvement, while with scores of 9-10 nearly all patients have nodal involvement.

STAGING

A commonly accepted clinical staging system based on digital rectal examination, acid phosphatase, bone survey or bone scan is shown in Table 11.3.

Table 11.3
Prostate Cancer Staging

Stage	Digital Exam	Acid Phos.	Bone Scan
A1	Tumor not detected	-	-
A2	Tumor not detected (more than 5 chips involved on TUR path)	-	-
B1	Tumor < 1.5 cm or involving only 1 lobe	-	-
B2	Tumor more than 1.5 cm or involving more than 1 lobe	-	-
C	Extracapsular tumor extention	+or-	-
D1	Any size tumor with pelvic nodal spread	+or-	-
D2	Any size tumor with distant nodal spread or bone or visceral metastases	+or-	+or-

WORK-UP

Physical examination with careful rectal exam, acid phosphatase (obtained prior to rectal exam), SMA-12 (in particular alkaline phosphatase), biopsy, bone scan, CBC, IVP and chest x-ray are recommended. Lymphangiogram or surgical lymph node sampling may be indicated to assess lymph node involvement.

TREATMENT AND RESULTS

A summary of results for commonly used treatments for prostate cancer is presented in Table 11.4.

Surgery: Radical prostatectomy consists of removal of the prostate including the prostatic capsule, urethra and seminal vesicles. This is effective treatment in localized B1 tumors where the degree of nodal involvement is not high (8-21%). Impotence occurs in 90-100% and urinary incontinence in 5-10% of patients following this procedure.

Radiotherapy: External beam radiation to doses of 6500-7000 rad to the prostate can effectively control local disease in patients with Stage A, B or C lesions. In patients with Stage C disease or when nodal disease is documented by lymphangiogram or node biopsy, the whole pelvis usually is initially treated to 4500 rad or more. Combined lymphadenectomy and whole pelvis radiation is not recommended due to a high incidence (greater than 25%) of penile, scrotal and leg edema. The role of prophylactic and therapeutic nodal irradiation is under investigation. Impotence occurs in 30-50% and incontinence in 5-10% of patients treated with high dose radiation. Biopsies of the prostate may be positive for over 18 months following radiation despite clinically inactive disease.

Interstitial radiation with I-125 prostatic implant has been used to treat localized prostatic cancer (Stage B1, B2 and small C). The efficacy requires a relatively small volume implant and homogenous I-125 seed distribution. Typically, an average peripheral dose of

15,000 to 18,000 rad is delivered to the prostate over one year. _In most institutions, this technique is performed only in the absence of pelvic nodal involvement._ Others have combined lymphadenectomy or pelvic irradiation with an implant when pelvic nodes are positive. The increase in morbidity from combined treatment is significant and the impact on survival is as yet undetermined. Local control is seen in 80-90% of implanted patients. About 25% of patients are impotent following radioactive implant of the prostate (though one institution reports less than 10%).

Table 11.4
A Summary of Results for Commonly Used Treatments for Prostate Cancer.

STAGE	TREATMENT	% LOCAL CONTROL	% SURVIVAL 5-YEAR	% SURVIVAL 10-YEAR
A1	Follow-up biopsy	100	95-100	95-100
A2	Prostate XRT	90		
B1	Radical prostatectomy versus		70	45
B2	Implant versus	90		
	External radiation to prostate & pelvis			
C	Pelvic & prostatic irradiation	85-90	40	30
D	Hormonal manipulation versus External radiation			

MORBIDITY

Acute

Diarrhea and dysuria often occur during prostatic irradiation and usually can be controlled with Lomotil and Pyridium respectively.

Chronic

The prostate is relatively resistant to radiation. Proctitis and cystitis occur in 10% of patients. Impotence occurs in 25-50% of patients treated with either implant or external beam radiation.

TESTICULAR MALIGNANCY

OVERVIEW

Management of malignant germ cell tumors of the testes has improved greatly through advances in treatment and a better understanding of the natural history afforded by lymphangiography, lymphadenectomy, radio-immunoassay for tumor markers and CT scanning. Seminomas are highly radiosensitive and can be cured in over 90% of patients with orchiectomy and radiation. Great improvement in the cure rate of advanced non-seminomatous testicular cancers (from less than 40% cure to over 80% cure) has resulted from the development of effective combination chemotherapy.

PATHOLOGY

Most testicular malignancies are of germ cell origin (See Table 11.5).

Table 11.5
Pathology of Testicular Malignancy

Germinal Origin (greater than 95% of patients)	%
Seminoma (typical, anaplastic, spermatocytic)	40
Non Seminoma (embryonal, teratomas, teratocarcinoma, choriocarcinoma)	55
Non Germinal Tumors	
Interstitial, gonadal, stromal	<5

CLINICAL FEATURES

Testicular cancer is the most common malignancy of males age 20-34. A testicular mass, with or without pain, is the most frequent presentation. Gynecomastia may be present with HCG secreting tumors.

Initial spread is along the lymphatics of the spermatic vein to the region of the renal pedicle. Retrograde spread then occurs to the nodes surrounding the vena cava and aorta. Subsequent spread may be through the thoracic duct to the left supraclavicular region or through transdiaphragmatic lymphatics to the mediastinum. Hematogenous metastases through direct vascular invasion may result in metastases to the lung, liver, brain or bone.

Patients with seminoma usually present with an early stage (65% of patients Stage I and 25% Stage II). Non-seminomatous tumors tend to be somewhat more advanced at presentation (45% Stage I, 35% Stage II, 25% Stage III).

STAGING

A TNM staging system is also in use.

Staging System (Based on clinical exam, orchiectomy, chest x-ray, lymphangiogram, IVP)

- I: Tumor confined to one testis. No evidence for spread beyond testis.
- II: Clinical or radiographic evidence of metastases to inguinal, iliac or para-aortic lymph nodes. No demonstrable visceral or supradiaphragmatic metastases.
  - IIA: Less than 5 cm tumor.
  - IIB: Greater than 5 cm tumor.
- III: Supradiaphragmatic nodal metastases.
- IV: Distant organ metastases.

WORK-UP

Work-up should include: (1) Routine - Physical examination, chest x-ray, CBC, IVP. (2) Bipedal lymphangiogram has 80-90% accuracy in detecting gross nodal involvement. The left renal hilar area, which is an important nodal drainage area, is not well opacified on lymphangiogram. (3) CT scan of the pelvis and abdomen complements the lymphangiogram in evaluating this area and determining the extent of retroperitoneal disease. (4) Serum alpha fetal protein (AFP) and human chorionic gonadotrophin (HCG). Approximately 90% of non-seminomatous tumors have elevations of either HCG or AFP. HCG is most commonly elevated with choriocarcinomas. The half-life of AFP is 5 days; the half-life of HCG is 1 day. (5) Diagnosis is made definitively at orchiectomy. Note: A trans-scrotal biopsy should not be performed due to the risk of seeding cancer into the scrotum.

TREATMENT AND RESULTS

SEMINOMA

Over 90% of patients with early stage disease (Stages I and II) are cured by inguinal orchiectomy and radiation therapy. Lymph node regions at risk for microscopic involvement are treated prophylactically with 2500 rad. Areas of gross disease are treated to

3500 rad. Advanced stage disease (Stages III and IV) or bulky disease (greater than 5 cm) may require initial chemotherapy with radiation given to residual disease sites (See Table 11.6).

Table 11.6
Treatment of Testicular Seminoma

STAGE	TREATMENT	5-YEAR SURVIVAL
I	2500 rad to "hockey stick" ie. homolateral iliacs and retroperitoneal nodes	98%
IIA	3500 rad to gross disease + 2500 rad to "hockey stick"; (mediastinum and left supraclavicular prophylaxis optional)	90%
IIB	Treatment as for IIA but boost gross disease to 4500 rad (versus treatment as for stage III and IV)	>60%
III & IV	Initial chemotherapy followed by radiation to residual disease	>60%

NON-SEMINOMATOUS TESTICULAR CANCER

Management of non-seminomatous tumors has improved greatly with the introduction of effective chemotherapy. There are many options available in treatment and the most efficacious method has not been determined.

Inguinal orhiectomy, which removes the testicular cancer, is usually followed by lymphadenectomy. Lymphadenectomy, though useful diagnostically in determining the presence of microscopic disease, is probably not therapeutic in most cases and is associated with significant morbidity including retrograde ejaculation or complete loss of ejaculatory capability in virtually all patients.

Lymphadenectomy followed by chemotherapy in node positive patients is a treatment regimen in common use. All chemotherapy regimens currently employ cis-platinum, bleomycin and vinblastine (VAB) with the possible addition of other agents (MTX, Adria, CTX). Stage I and II non-seminomatous tumors have also been treated with orchiectomy and lymphadenectomy alone with chemotherapy given if recurrent disease manifests. This approach requires close follow-up with bimonthly chest x-rays and serum markers for at least two years; 85-95% cure is expected. Lymphadenectomy or tumor resection should be combined with chemotherapy in the treatment of advanced disease (bulky Stage II, and stage III and IV). Cure rates for advanced disease appear to be in the range of 60-80% or greater.

Radiation can control microscopic and occasionally gross nonseminomatous cancer, but doses used must be higher than for seminoma (4000-4500 rad). Survival after radiation for clinical Stage I and Stage IIA disease without lymphadenopathy is over 80%; therefore, this is a viable alternative for early stage non-seminomas. Relapse can be detected early by use of serum markers. Chemotherapy may salvage about 50% of radiotherapy failures. More advanced stages are poorly controlled with radiation alone (35% survival).

MORBIDITY (from radiation)

Acute

Doses of 2500 rad to the "hockey stick" field have few acute side effects - possibly nausea, fatigue, diarrhea.

Chronic

Virtually no chronic effects are seen with 2500 rad to 3400 rad to "hockey stick". Care must be taken to limit the dose to the kidneys.

Radiation effect on the testicle

The testis is very sensitive to radiation and doses of less than 100 rad may cause oligospermia. Doses of up to 600 rad may cause temporary sterility.

Higher doses may result in permanent sterility. Depletion of sperm is seen soon after doses of greater than 400 rad since spermatocytes are killed directly (interphase death). Lower doses effect spermatogonia and oligospermia usually is not seen until nearly seven weeks following radiation; aspermia requires another three weeks.

Fortunately, the majority of patients treated for testicular cancer will not require scrotal irradiation. Therefore, the scattered dose to the remaining testicle from the "hockey stick" radiation is very low and should not result in sterility. Scrotal irradiation may be required when a transcrotal biopsy has been performed

REFERENCES

1. Holland JM: Cancer of the kidney - natural history and staging. Cancer 32:1030-1042,1973.
2. Mohiuddin M, Strong GH, Mulholland SG: Combined pre- and postoperative adjuvant radio-therapy for bladder cancer. Urology 19:135-138, 1982.
3. vanderWerf Messing B et al: Carcinoma of the urinary bladder treated by pre-operative irradiation followed by simple cystectomy. Int J Rad Onc Bio Phys 8:1839-55, 1982.
4. vanderWerf Messing B: Carcinoma of the urinary bladder treated by interstital radium implant. I J Rad Onc Bio Phys 4:373-378, 1978.
5. Nelson RP: New concepts in staging and follow-up of bladder cancer. Urology 21:105-110, 1983.
6. Bagsha M, Pistenbma D et al: External beam radiation therapy in primary carcinoma of the prostate. Cancer 36:723-728, 1975.
7. Hilaris B et al: Behavioral patterns of prostate adenocarcinoma following I-125 implant and pelvic node dissection. I J Rad Onc Bio Phys 2:631-637, 1977.
8. Klein LA: Prostatic carcinoma. N Eng J Med 300:824-833,1979.
9. Einhorn L, Donohue J: Cis-pt., vinblastine and bleomycin combination chemotherapy in disseminated testicular cancer. Ann Int Med 87:293-298, 1977.
10. Maier J, Mihemeyer: Carcinoma of the testis. Cancer 39:901-986,1977.
11. Shipley, WU: Personal communication.

Chapter 12

Gynecologic Cancer

UTERINE CERVIX

OVERVIEW

Invasive cervical carcinoma can be effectively treated with radiation therapy even when relatively advanced. A combination of external and intracavitary radiation is frequently used in order to maximize the dose delivered to the central and parametrial disease as well as to treat pelvic lymph nodes. Surgery can be used in selected early cases alone or in combination with radiation.

PATHOLOGY

Grossly, cervical cancers are of three distinct types: ulcerating, exophytic and nodular. Most frequently they arise from the posterior cervical lip, followed in frequency by the cervical canal and anterior lip.

Microscopically, approximately 90% of cervical cancers are squamous cell, usually moderate to poorly differentiated. Ten percent are other histologies, including adenocarcinoma (includes clear cell), oat cell and glassy cell (a variant of poorly differentiated squamous). In a high proportion of instances the sequence of dysplasia to carcinoma in situ to infiltrating carcinoma may occur. Carcinoma in situ usually develops at the squamo-columnar junction and involves the whole depth of the epithelium. Microinvasive carcinoma invades the epithelial-stromal junction to a maximum of 3 to 5 mm.

CLINICAL FEATURES

The number of invasive cancers is declining. There is an increased risk of cervical cancer among women of low socioeconomic groups, those who begin sexual activity at an early age, and those with numerous sexual partners. Herpes simplex virus (type II) has been associated with cervical cancer.

Patients with cervical cancer frequently present with vaginal discharge, bleeding or pelvic pain. Anemia is frequently present. Local spread occurs through three major routes: 1) inferiorly into the vagina, 2) laterally into the parametrium and 3) superiorly into the body of the uterus. Extension into the uterus does not affect the stage but is associated with a worse prognosis. Extension into the bladder or rectum may occur with advanced disease. Pelvic and para-aortic nodes become increasingly ivolved with higher stage disease (See Table 12.1).

Table 12.1
Lymph Node Involvement versus Stage

Stage	% Positive Pelvic Nodes	% Positive Para-aortic Nodes
I_a <3 mm	< 1	---
I_a 3-5 mm	5-8	---
I_b	15	5
II	33	15-20
III	50	30-40

STAGING

Stage 0: Carcinoma in situ, intraepithelial carcinoma.

Stage I: Carcinoma strictly confined to cervix.

Ia: Microinvasive carcinoma (early stromal invasion of less than 3-5 mm).

Ib: All other cases of stage I; occult cancer should be marked occ.

Stage II: Extension beyond cervix, but not to pelvic sidewall. Vaginal involvement, but not to distal third.

IIa: No obvious parametrial involvement.
IIb: Obvious parametrial involvement.
Stage III: Extension to pelvic sidewall and/or to lower third of vagina. All cases with hydronephrosis or a nonfunctioning kidney are included, unless they are known to be due to another cause.
IIIa: No extension to pelvic sidewall.
IIIb: Extension to pelvic sidewall and/or hydronephrosis.
Stage IV: Extension beyond true pelvis or clinical involvement of bladder or rectal mucosa. (Bullous edema of the bladder mucosa is insufficient for classification as Stage IV).
IVa: Extension to adjacent organs.
IVb: Metastases to distant organs.

WORK-UP

Early asymptomatic disease may be detected by routine Pap smear. Current recommendations for Pap smear are that asymptomatic women 20 years of age and older and those under 20 who are sexually active should have a Pap smear annually for two years, then once every three years until age 65.

Routine evaluation for suspected cervical cancer should include exam under anesthesia with cervical biopsy and fractional D&C. Also IVP, cystoscopy, proctoscopy, chest x-ray, CBC & serum chemistries (SMA-12) are required for staging purposes, though cystosocpy and proctoscopy have a low yield for early disease. T/C: bone scan & liver scan for advanced disease.

Lymphangiogram and abdominal-pelvic CT scans may be of value in detecting pelvic or para-aortic adenopathy but cannot be used in staging. Radiographically suspicious lymph nodes may be evaluated by a skinny needle aspiration biopsy, perhaps eliminating the need for laparotomy. The value of pretreatment lymph node sampling (particularly para-aortic nodes) by an extraperitoneal or transabdominal approach is being studied.

TREATMENT AND RESULTS

Treatment must be individualized on the basis of the patient's stage, age, medical condition and presence of contraindications, as well as physician availability. Radiation is the treatment of choice for most patients; however, selected early cases may be managed surgically. Radiation is contraindicated in the presence of severe pelvic inflammatory disease.

A general outline of important surgical and radiotherapeutic considerations is presented below:

Surgery

Cervical conization may be used in patients with *in situ* (Stage 0) cancer who are desirous of having children. Otherwise, *in situ* carcinoma and early Stage I_A (less than 3 mm of invasion) tumors may be treated with total abdominal hysterectomy and vaginal cuff resection.

A *Wertheim radical hysterectomy* may be used in patients with Stage IB disease and selected patients with Stage IIA disease. It consists of removal of the uterus, tubes, ovaries, broad ligament and parametrium, wide vaginal cuff and regional lymph nodes. Ovaries are often spared in young patients.

An *extrafascial abdominal hysterectomy* may be used in combination with preoperative radiation in some patients with Stage IB "barrel shaped" cervix or with extension of cervical cancer into the endometrium. Combined surgery and radiation offer improved local control over radiation alone in these selected cases with large central disease but no parametrial extension.

Radiation Therapy

The role of curative surgery diminishes once tumor has spread beyond the confines of the cervix and vaginal fornices. Intracavitary radiation for central pelvic disease and external beam radiation for lateral parametrial and pelvic nodal disease may then be utilized (See Chapter 1).

Intracavitary Radiation: Radioactive isotopic sources, usually cesium-137 or radium, can be introduced directly into the uterine cavity and vaginal fornices with speciäl applicators. An applicator usually consists of a tandem, which holds sources within the uterine cavity, and colpostats, which hold sources in the vaginal fornices. A Fletcher-Suit afterloading applicator is one of the several types of tandem and colpostat applicators used.

The dose delivered by intracavitary radiation may be expressed in terms of milligram-hours or rads. Milligram-hour dosage is calculated by determining the number of milligrams of radium or radium-equivalent material inserted and multiplying that by the number of hours of insertion (e.g. if 6 sources, each 10 mg radium equivalent, are left in place for 50 hours, the mg-hour dosage is 60 mg x 50 hours = 3000 mg-hours). Standardized source loading, applicator positioning and long experience in the use of the mg-hr system makes it widely accepted.

There is also extensive experience with prescribing the rad dose to a point. The rad dose is determined from the dose rate (rad/hour) multiplied times the number of hours the sources are in place. The dose rate to a point or a number of points from a particular source arrangement can be calculated. Adjustments in the strength or positioning of the sources can then be made to yield a selected dose rate to a point or number of points. Points of interest usually include the maximum rectal and bladder dose as well as the dose to two standard pelvic points, point A and point B. Point A is located 2 cm cephalad from the lateral fornix and 2 cm lateral to the uterine canal. Anatomically it represents the medial parametrium, approximately where the ureter and uterine artery cross. Point B is 3 cm lateral to point A and approximates the region of the obturator node. Due to variations in the anatomy of this region, particularly those caused by tumor, these points may not strictly correspond to the anatomic structures indicated.

External beam radiation: External pelvic irradiation is used in conjunction with intracavitary radiation when extension into the parametria or pelvic lymph node involvement are present or suspected. The amount of external beam radiation delivered and the timing of its administration relative to intracavitary radiation is individualized. For example, the presence of an exophytic cancer which distorts the cervix would preclude successful placement of intracavitary radiation initially. External beam radiation would be administered first and, after significant regression of disease, could be followed by intracavitary radiation. Advanced tumors require relatively more external beam radiation due to the inability of central radioisotope sources to effectively irradiate disease in the lateral parametrium.

External para-aortic irradiation may be used in addition to pelvic radiation when para-aortic disease is confirmed or suspected. Though radiation can successfully sterilize microscopic disease, its value in the treatment of gross disease is limited since the tolerance of surrounding organs (bowel, kidney) preclude delivery of high doses to the para-aortic region.

Chemotherapy

Chemotherapy may be of value in the treatment of disseminated cervical cancer and in locally recurrent cancer not amenable to further surgery or radiation. There is no standard chemotherapy regimen for cervical cancer and several investigational protocols are underway. A number of single agents produce response rates of about 20% and combination chemotherapy responses range from 10% to 50%.

Chemotherapy is also under investigation for adjuvant use in patients with high common iliac or para-aortic nodal involvement since they have a high likelihood for having disseminated disease.

Table 12.2 lists treatment options for various stages of disease along with relative five-year survival.

Table 12.2
Treatment and Survival in Cervical Cancer

Stage	Treatment Options	5-Year Survival
0	1. Conization in young desirous of children 2. TAH 3. Intracavitary radiation	100%
Ia (<3mm)	1. TAH 2. Intracavitary radiation	100%
Ia (3-5 mm)	1. Radical hysterectomy 2. External + intracavitary radiation	95-100%
Ib	1. Radical hysterectomy 2. External + intracavitary radiation 3. See * below	90%
IIa	1. External + intracavitary radiation 2. Radical hysterectomy in selected patients 3. See * below	80%
IIb	1. External + intracavitary radiation	60%
III	1. External + intracavitary radiation	30-45%
IV	1. External radiation alone or with intracavitary radiation 2. Anterior or posterior exenteration ±radiation in selected cases 3. Chemotherapy for disseminated disease	5-20%

*Radiotherapy followed by extrafascial hysterectomy in patients with "barrel shaped" cervix or uterine extension.

Recurrent disease usually manifests early. Over 70% of patients who develop recurrent cancer do so within 2 years of treatment. The majority of recurrences are distant metastases to lung or bone though nearly one-third will be in the pelvis. The triad of low back pain, lower extremity edema and an abnormal IVP usually signifies locally recurrent disease. (Pap smears may be useful in helping determine local recurrence but it is important to note that they are usually abnormal for three to four months following radiation and therefore are of little value during that period.) Occasionally, locally recurrent disease may be amenable to curative surgery or radiation. Chemotherapy is used for most disseminated cervical cancer. Palliative radiation may be of value for symptomatic bone metastases, spinal cord compression, mediastinal compression, etc.

MORBIDITY

Acute

During pelvic radiation, patients may experience fatigue, diarrhea and cystitis. Anorexia and nausea may also occur if the para-aortic region is also treated.

Chronic

The cervix can tolerate doses of 20,000 rad without necrosis. Severe late complications, such as chronic cystitis, proctosigmoiditis and small bowel damage following radiation are generally seen in less than 10% of patients treated. Fistulae occasionally occur with advanced disease. The risk of late small bowel complications, (enteritis and obstruction), following pelvic radiation is increased in patients with diabetes or hypertension, and especially when both are present. Pelvic radiation following radical hysterectomy and pelvic lymph node dissection may carry an increased risk of late complictions. Para-aortic radiation, particularly following surgical evaluation of para-aortic nodes, can result in severe late bowel complications in over one-third of patients treated.

ENDOMETRIUM

OVERVIEW

Although endometrial cancer is the most frequent gynecologic malignancy, it results in far fewer deaths than ovarian or cervical cancer. The relatively good prognosis is due to the large percentage of patients who present with early disease and the existence of effective treatment modalities for early disease, namely surgery and radiation therapy. Advanced stages are managed with radiation alone and the outcome is less favorable.

PATHOLOGY

Grossly, endometrial carcinomas are flat but occasionally may be pedunulated. They may be preceded by endometrial polyps.

Microscopically, carcinomas of the endometrium are classified into three major groups: adenocarcinoma, adenoacanthomas and adenosquamous.

Adenocarcinoma (70%): 60% Grade I, 20% Grade II. Adenoacanthoma (20%): Adenocarcinoma with squamous metaplasia. Adenosquamous (10%): Squamous component is malignant but the prognosis is related to degree of differentiation of the adenocarcinoma.

It is not clear as to whether endometrial hyperplasia gives rise to carcinoma but microscopically they are frequently associated.

Sarcomas of the uterus also occur and can be divided as follows: Pure (one cell line),mixed (more than one cell line), homologous (cells usually found in uterus), and heterologous (cells not usually found in the uterus).

CLINICAL FEATURES

Adenocarcinoma of the endometrium occurs most frequently in the postmenopausal age group. Prior use of exogenous estrogen results in an increased risk of endometrial cancer. Associated medical problems include obesity, diabetes mellitus and hypertension.

The presenting symptom of endometrial cancer is usually vaginal bleeding. Pain is not an early symptom. Urinary symptoms and constipation may occur with advanced tumors. The disease tends to remain localized in the uterus. Initial spread is into the myometrium. Extension inferiorly into the cervix is associated with increased incidence of pelvic nodal disease. The incidence of nodal disease is dependent on stage, grade and depth of myometrial invasion (see Table 12.3). Para-aortic nodal spread, peritoneal seeding and distant metastases may also occur.

Table 12.3
Positive Pelvic Nodes (% PPN)

Depth of Myometrial Invasion	%PPN	Stage	%PPN	Grade	%PPN
inner 1/3	10%	I	10	1	5
middle 1/3	20%	II	35	2	10
outer 1/3	45%			3	25-45%

STAGING

Stage 0: Carcinoma in situ.
Stage I: Confined to uterus.
Ia: Uterine length 8 cm or less
Ib: Uterine length greater than 8 cm
Recommended: Subgrouping stage I cases by histologic grade.
G1: Highly differentiated carcinoma.
G2: Moderately differentiated carcinoma.
G3: Predominately solid or undifferentiated carcinoma.
Stage II: Extension to cervix (Corpus et colli)
Stage III: Extrauterine extension but not outside the true pelvis
Stage IV: Extrapelvic extension or involvement of bladder or rectal mucosa or metastases.

WORK-UP

A fractional D&C and cervical biopsy, exam under anesthesia, cystoscopy, CBC and SMA-12, IVP, chest x-ray, proctoscopy and BE are accepted by FIGO in establishing the clinical stage for endometiral carcinoma. A bone scan and liver scan (among others) may be indicated for advanced disease.

TREATMENT AND RESULTS

Stage I: Surgery, including TAH and BSO, is indicated. Patients with deep myometrial invasion or high grade tumors are given adjuvant radiotherapy to prevent local failure. Approximately 4500-5000 rad may be given either pre or postoperatively. Radiation reduces vaginal apex recurrence from 10-20% to less than 5%. Use of aggressive radiotherapy alone is often successful in inoperable patients, but there is a likely a 10-15% decrease in survival compared to surgery alone.

Stage II: Regardless of grade or depth of invasion, when cervical involvement is present, combined surgery and radiation is usually indicated due to the risk of vaginal and pelvic nodal disease. Preoperative radiotherapy, either external beam alone (4500-5000 rad) or in combination with intracavitary radiation, followed by TAH and BSO 4 weeks after completion of radiation is a successful management scheme in common use. Postoperative external beam pelvic radiation to 5000 rad may be used instead of pre-op radiation. Combined surgery and radiation results in a 5-year survival of over 75% in Stage II endometrial carcinoma.

Stage III and IVA: When disease has extended into the pelvis, cure rates drop to 10-15%. These patients are technically inoperable and radiation alone is usually indicated. Occasionally, selected patients may receive preoperative radiation and surgery. Patients with clinical stage II, pathologic stage III disease, particularly when only tubes and ovaries are involved outside the uterus , fare better than other stage III patients (over 40% 5-year surival). Though local failure remains a significant problem, distant spread out of the pelvis is often encountered. Use of adjuvant chemotherapy is being explored. Hormonal treatment with synthetic progestational agents may be of value since 30-40% response rates may be obtained in patients treated for recurrent disease, with a prolongation in survival noted amongst responders.

A summary of the results of currently used treatment schemes is presented in Table 12.4.

Table 12.4
Treatment and Results in Endometrial Cancer

Stage	Treatment	5-Yr. Survival
I	Radiation alone	65-70%
	Surgery alone	75-80%
	Radiation + surgery*	90%
II	Radiation alone	55%
	Surgery alone	60%
	Radiation + surgery	75-80%
III, IVA	Radiation alone	10-15%

*used in patients with deeply invasive or high grade tumors

Treatment of Pelvic Failures: About 1/2 of patients who fail after surgical treatment alone will fail in the pelvis. One half of these pelvic failures occur in the vagina. Twenty to 40% of pelvic failures can be salvaged by radiation therapy.

Sarcomas are treated primarily surgically. Leimyosarcomas are associated with a better survival than other histologies. Adjuvant postoperative radiotherapy is recommended for most sarcomas (except perhaps Stage I leiomyosarcomas) to diminish pelvic failures. Advanced endometrial stromal sarcomas and some mixed mesodermal tumors may respond to radiation alone. Since distant metastases (lung, liver) are the most common site of failure, systemic chemotherapy is important in the comprehensive treatment of uterine sarcomas. The overall 5 year survival ranges from nearly 60% for Stage I and 40% for Stage II to virtually no survivors with Stage III and IV disease.

MORBIDITY

Acute and chronic complications are similar to those encountered in the treatment of cervical cancer. The risk factors associated with endometrial carcinoma, such as diabetes, obesity, hypertension may make patients medically inoperable or delay postoperative recovery.

OVARY

OVERVIEW

Despite the fact that ovarian cancer is less common than cervical or endometrial cancer, it produces more deaths than both combined. Surgery is essential, both diagnostically, to determine sites of involvement, and therapeutically, to resect gross deposits, so that postsurgically only minimal residual disease is left to be treated with chemotherapy or radiation.

PATHOLOGY

Since the ovary is histologically a very complex structure it may give rise to a variety of tumors. Aproximately 80% of ovarian cancers are of epithelial origin (serous 45%; mucinous 10%; endometroid 15%; mixed type, clear type and Brenner tumors < 10%). About 10% of ovarian malignancies are of germ cell origin (dysgerminoma, endodermal sinus tumors, choriocarcinoma, embryonal teratocarcinomas). Tumors of stromal origin account for about 5% (granulosa cell, Stertoli-Leydig cell). Tumors of undeterminate origin comprise 5-10%.

Since serous and mucinous carcinomas are frequently encountered ovarian malignancies, it is important to know their distinguishing pathologic features. These are presented in Table 12.5.

Table 12.5
Distinguishing Pathologic Features of Serous and Mucinous Ovarian Carcinoma.

	Serous Cystadenocarcinoma	Mucinous Cystadenocarcinoma
Frequency (% of all ovarian malignancies)	45%	15%
Ratio of benign to malignant type (i.e. adenoma/carcinoma)	1/1	9/1
% Bilateral	50%	20%
Microscopic	cuboidal, cilia often present, psammoma bodies frequent	high columnar, no cilia, no psammoma bodies

Grade is an important prognostic indicator and will be discussed later. Tumors of borderline malignant potential do not infiltrate the stroma of the ovary but may spread beyond the ovary and seed the peritoneal surfaces.

CLINICAL FEATURES

The incidence of ovarian cancer peaks in the 40-60 age group. Risk factors include low parity and infertility. Since early disease rarely causes symptoms, most patients present with advanced disease. Symptoms of nausea, mass or pressure in the pelvis and increased abdominal girth are common.

Four modes of spread are common: 1) lymphatic, 2) direct extension, 3) peritoneal seeding and 4) hematogenous.

Lymphatic spread occurs to the pelvic lymph nodes and also directly to para-aortic nodes via lymphatics along the infundibulopelvic ligament. Direct extension through the capsule may result in involvement of adjacent pelvic structres: tubes, uterus, bladder, rectum. Peritoneal seeding may also occur whenever capsular penetration is noted. Seeding may give rise to tumor deposits anywhere in the abdomen, but the diaphragm is at particularly high risk. Hematogenous spread occurs to lung, liver and bone.

Important prognostic factors include stage, degree of differentiation and completeness of resection. The majority of patients felt to be clinically Stage I or II will be found to have more advanced disease at surgery. If complete resection with only minimal residual disease (less than 2 cm) cannot be accomplished, survival is decreased by more than 50%.

Borderline malignant tumors have a better prognosis than common epithelial ovarian cancers and results should be reported separately.

STAGING

T Classification

Stage I: Growth limited to ovaries
- IA: Limited to one ovary; no ascites
  - IAi: Capsule intact
  - IAii: Capsule ruptured and/or tumor on external surface
- IB: Growth limited to both ovaries; no ascites
  - IBi: Capsule intact
  - IBii: Capsule ruptured and/or tumor on external surface
- IC: Either IA or IB with ascites, or positive peritoneal washings.

Stage II: Growth involving one or both ovaries with pelvic extension
- IIA: Extension to uterus and/or tubes
- IIB: Extension to other pelvic tissues
- IIC: Either IIA or IIB with ascites or positive peritoneal washings

Stage III: Extrapelvic intraperitoneal metastases and/or positive retroperitoneal nodes. Tumor limited to pelvis with biopsy-proven small bowel or omental extension

Stage IV: Distant metastases, liver metastases, or cytologically positive pleural fluid

WORK-UP

The differential diagnosis of a pelvic mass is large and includes amongst others ovarian cysts, endometriosis, pelvic inflammatory disease, ectopic pregnancy, diverticular disease and carcinoma of the colon. Initial evaluation should include a careful history and physical exam, chest x-ray, IVP, barium enema, CBC, SMA-12, and proctoscopy. A CT scan or ultrasound of pelvis, examination under anesthesia with fractional dilatation and curettage, cytology and lymphangiogram are often done subsequently.

Laparotomy and surgical exploration are essential and should include when possible:

1. TAH and BSO
2. Inspection and biopsy of liver, diaphragm, para-aortic nodes
3. Abdominal and pelvic washings for cytology
4. Debulking of gross disease to minimum (preferably less than .5 cm)
5. Areas of residual disease should be clipped
6. Omentectomy (to remove possible present or potential site of disease spread)

TREATMENT AND RESULTS

OVARIAN CARCINOMAS

Surgery: A TAH and BSO with complete or maximal tumor resection and diagnostic procedures as outlined above are indicated in all operable patients. (Patients with a stage IA lesion of borderline malignant potential represents one exception where less surgery may be advisable). The volume of residual tumor remains an extremely important factor in determing response to further treatment.

Chemotherapy: Adjuvant chemotherapy includes single agent and multiagent treatment regimens. There is some evidence that with minimal postsurgical residual disease multidrug chemotherapy may be better than single agent chemotherapy. Significant responses to chemotherapy may also be seen with advanced stage III and IV disease. In general, the response to chemotherapy may be affected by the presence of minimal residual disease (< 1.5 to 2.0 cm) at initial surgery, tumor grade, prior chemotherapy exposure, performance status and completeness of restaging.

Radiation Therapy: *Total abdominal radiation* (which includes the entire peritoneal surface and diaphragm) may improve survival of patients with completely resected disease or minimal residual disease. Radiotherapeutic techniques require sophisticated treatment planning since G.I., liver and kidney tolerance must be respected. Abdominal radiation may be accomplished by giving low daily doses to the whole abdomen, or a *moving strip technique* of total abdominal radiation. With this technique high dose fraction radiation is given to a strip across the abdomen, and the strip is advanced daily down the abdomen in an attempt to improve radiobiologic effectiveness and decrease toxicity of external beam radiation. *Intraperitoneal P-32* or radiogold has been used to treat suspected microscopic disease within the peritoneal cavity when free flow of peritoneal fluid can be demonstrated.

DYSGERMINOMA

This tumor is highly sensitive to radiotherapy. Radiotherapy is indicated in all patients with extracapsular extension and no evidence of extralymphatic metastases. Radiation is usually directed to the affected lymph node regions plus the next unaffected nodal echelon or the whole abdomen. A careful pathologic search for mixed tumor elements should be made since, if found, more aggressive management with inclusion of chemotherapy is in order.

The overall survival for dysgerminoma is about 85% following surgery and radiation. About one-third of patients with advanced disease with distant metastases or with recurrent tumors may be sucessfully treated by combination chemotherapy.

MORBIDITY

Acute

Total abdominal radiation is associated with *nausea*, *vomiting* and *diarrhea*. *Myelosuppression* severe enough to warrant interruption of therapy occurs in up to 20% of patients.

Chronic

Chronic enteritis requiring surgical intervention occurs rarely. Radiation hepatitis and nephritis should not occur if care is taken in treatment planning to block or limit the dose to the liver and kidneys.

Effect of radiation on the ovaries: A single dose of 200 rad may produce temporary arrest of menses. Nearly 2000 rad is required to produce permanent cessation of menstruation. The radiation effect on the ovary is dependent on the patient's age, with older patients being less sensitive than younger patients.

VAGINA

OVERVIEW

Vaginal cancer by definition can have no cervical or vulvar involvement. These tumors are quite rare and account for less than 2% of gynecologic malignancies. Vaginal cancers include squamous cell carcinoma, which arise in elderly women (median age of 62), and adenocarcinomas, frequently seen in young women exposed to DES in utero (median age of 19).

Radiotherapy is effective in the mangement of this disease. When advanced disease is present, interstitial and intracavitary radiation is often required along with external beam radiotherapy.

Survival is quite good for early lesions without significant pelvic spread (60 to 80%). When disease is adherent to the pelvic wall or adjacent organs are involved, survival drops to about 25%

VULVA

OVERVIEW

Vulvar cancers, usually squamous cell carcinomas, are seen in elderly females. They may arise from areas of vulvar dysplasia. Treatment of vulvar cancers is primarly surgical. Inguinal or pelvic nodal irradiation to 4500-5000 rad may be used to treat nodes at risk for microscopic disease with less morbidity than extensive nodal dissections. Higher doses of radiation to the perineum, inguinal region or pelvis are poorly tolerated and should be avoided.

An overall survival of 75% is seen in patients with negative inguinal nodes and 41% in patients with positive nodes. When pelvic nodes are positive, survival is only 20%.

REFERENCES

1. Bush R, Allt W, Beal F, et al: Treatment of epithelial carcinoma of the ovary: Operation, irradiation and chemotherapy. Am J Ob Gyne 127:692-704, 1977.
2. Marcial V: Carcinoma of the cervix. Cancer 39: 943-958, 1977.
3. Morrow C, DiSaia P, Townsend D: Current management of endometrial carcinoma. Ob and Gyne. 43:399-405, 1973.
4. Montraverdi R, Bardawil W, Lochan D, et al: Uterine sarcomas: an analysis of 69 patients. I J Rad Bio Phys 7:917-922, 1981.
5. Chung C, Stryker J, Nahas W, et al: Analysis of residual disease following pre-operative radiotherapy versus initial surgery in endometrial carcinoma. I J Rad Bio Phys 8:213-219, 1982.
6. Abayomi O, Dritschilo A, Emami B, et al: The value of "routine tests" in the staging evaluation of gynecologic malignancies. I J Rad Bio Phys: 8:241-245, 1982.
7. Piver M.: Optimal surgical therapy in stage I and II ovarian malignancies. I J Rad Bio Phys 8: 247-250, 1982.
8. Dalley V: The role of radiotherapy and chemotherapy in treatment of cancer of the ovary. I J Rad Bio Phys 8:251-256, 1982.
9. Hamburger A, Fletcher G: Is surgical evaluation of the para-aortic nodes prior to irradiation of benefit in carcinoma of the cervix? I J Rad Bio Phys 8:151-154, 1982.
10. Danoff B, McDay J, Louka M, et al: Stage III endometrial carcinoma. Analysis of patterns of failure and therapeutic implications. I J Rad Bio Phys 6:1491-1496, 1980.

11. Hintz B, Kagan A, Chan P, et al: Radiation tolerance of the vaginal mucosa. I J Rad Bio Phys 6:711-716, 1980.
12. Malkasian G, Decker D, Mussey E, et al: Radiation therapy in carcinoma of the vagina. Am J Ob Gyne 110:15-21, 1971.
13. Perez C, Aneson A, Dehner L, et al: Radiation therapy in carcinoma of the vagina. Ob Gyne 44:862-872, 1974.
14. Franklin E, Rutledge F: Prognostic factors in epidermoid carcinoma of the vulva. Ob Gyne 37:892-901, 1971.
15. Brody S: Clinical aspects of dysgerminoma of the ovary. Am J Rad 56:209-230, 1961.
16. Dembo AJ, van Dyke J, Tapp B, et al: Whole abdominal irradiation by a moving-strip technique for patients with ovarian cancer. I J Rad Bio Phys 5:1922-1942, 1979.
17. Bast R, Klug T, St. John E: A radioimmunoassay using a monoclonal antibody to monitor the course of epithelial ovarian cancer. N Eng J Med 309:883-887, 1983.

Chapter 13

Soft Tissue Sarcomas

OVERVIEW

These tumors of mesenchymal origin involve the connective tissue of the extremities, torso and viscera. They are relatively rare tumors with an approximate incidence of 4800 new cases per year. Combined-modality treatment results in a high percentage of local cures with the potential advantages of decreased morbidity and preservation of function compared to radial surgery or radiation alone.

PATHOLOGY

Table 13.1 lists the presumed tissues of origin for the various soft tissue sarcomas and the incidence range in the literature. The wide variation in incidence reflects not only case selection but also the difficulty that pathologists often experience in sub-classifying these tumors. Since 1972, malignant fibrous histiocytoma has been reported and has become increasingly recognized. Histologic grade correlates with survival and has been incorporated in the staging system. Grade for grade, there does not appear to be major differences in the clinical behavior of the various histologic subtypes of soft tissue sarcoma.

Malignant fibrous histiocytomas (MFH) can occur in three major forms: fibroblast, histiocytic and pleomorphic with the pleomorphic variety most likely to disseminate distantly. Fibrosarcomas may be subclassified as fibrocystic, fibroblastic and pleomorphic with the latter two being high grade. Liposarcomas may be well differentiated, myxoid, lipoblastic, fibroblastic and pleomorphic. The myxoid and well differentiated varieties are low grade and carry more favorable prognoses. They are relatively radiosensitive and may regress rapidly after even low doses of radiation. Rhabdomyosarcomas present in three histologic forms: pleomorphic, alveolar and embryonal.

Pleomorphic rhabdomyosarcoma was the form most frequently reported in adults but most of these tumors are presently classified as MFH. The alveolar and embryonal rhabdomyosarcomas are tumors of childhood and will be discussed further in Chapter 15.

Table 13.1
Presumed Tissues of Origin for the Various Soft Tissue Sarcomas and the Incidence Range

Histology	Tissue or cell origin	Incidence Range (%)
Rhabdomyosarcoma	Striated muscle	5.0-30.0
Liposarcoma	Adipose	11.5-27.6
Fibrosarcoma	Fibrous	1.7-44.0
Malignant Fibrous Histiocytoma	Histiocyte	0-20.4
Neurogenic Sarcoma	Neural	0-19.3
Synovial Sarcoma	Synovium	0.8-14.1
Leiomyosarcoma	Smooth muscle	2.4-11.3
Mesenchymoma	Primitive mesenchyme	0-0.3
Unclassified	Uncertain	0-36.4
Angiosarcoma	Vascular	0-4.8
Alveolar Soft Parts Sarcoma	Paraganglia?	Rare
Lymphangiosarcoma	Lymphatic	Rare
Dermatofibrosarcoma Protuberans	Perineural fibroblast	Rare

CLINICAL FEATURES

Soft tissue sarcomas can occur at any age, although peak incidences are noted in childhood and the fifth decade of life. There is no sex predilection. These tumors present as mass lesions which progress in size and cause local pain. Lower extremity lesions account for 40% of these tumors, Retroperitoneal sarcomas account for 15% and often present as huge tumors with obstructive symptoms of the GI or GU tracts.

The incidence of head and neck sarcomas varies from 5-15%, and upper extremity lesions account for 10-25%. Soft tissue sarcomas have a propensity to metastasize hematogenously, particularly to lung. Regional lymph nodes metastasis may also occur in 10-15% of patients with rhabdomyosarcoma, MFH and synovial sarcomas.

STAGING

The AJC staging system, which incorporates histologic grading, is presented below. The prognostic significance of the stage grouping has been demonstrated in large retrospective studies.

TNM Classification

Primary Tumor (T)

- TX Minimum requirements to assess the primary tumor cannot be met.
- T0 No demonstrable tumor
- T1 Tumor 5 cm or less in diameter
- T2 Tumor more than 5 cm in diameter
- T3 Clear radiographic evidence of destruction of cortical bone, with invasion; histopathologic confirmation of invasion of major artery or nerve

Nodal Involement (N)

- NX Minimum requirements to assess the regional nodes cannot be met
- N0 No histologically verified regional lymph node metastasis
- N1 Histologically verified regional lymph node metastasis

Distant Metastasis (M)

- MX Minimum requirements to assess the presence of distant metastasis cannot be met
- M0 No (known) distant metastasis
- M1 Distant metastasis present

Histologic Grade of Malignancy (G)

- G1 Low
- G2 Moderate
- G3 High

Stage Grouping

Stage IA	G1,T1,N0,M0
Stage IB	G1,T2,N0,M0
Stage IIA	G2,T1,N0,M0
Stage IIB	G2,T2,N0,M0
Stage IIIA	G3,T1,N0,M0
Stage IIIB	G3,T1-2,N0,M0
Stage IIIC	G T1-2,N1,M0
Stage IVA	any G,T3,N0-1
Stage IVB	any G,T or N,M1

WORK-UP

All unexplained soft tissue masses, which are persistent, enlarging or painful should be biopsied using needle, incisional, or for small lesions, excisional techniques. The proper placement of biopsy incisions is of great importance so as not to compromise later surgical or radiotherapeutic management. Once a tissue type and grade has been established, work-up should be directed to evaluate local extent and rule out the presence of distant metastatic disease. Pretreatment evaluation by clinicians with appropriate surgical, radiotherapuetic and chemotherapeutic expertise optimizes management. CT scanning and arteriography are helpful in evaluating local extent. Chest x-ray and whole lung tomography or thoracic CT scanning are indicated to evaluate for lung metastases.

TREATMENT AND RESULTS

The management of soft tissue sarcomas is similar regardless of histology and will, therefore, be discussed in general terms.

Surgery and Radiation

Resectable extremity lesions have traditionally been treated by radical surgery including amputation and radical soft part resection. Radical surgery will achieve local control in 70-90% of patients. Local exision alone has a recurrence rate of up to 80%. The failure of less radical surgery to yield local cure is due to the persistence of microscopic tumor in the surgical bed. Control of microscopic residua by postoperative irradiation along with preservation of function and anatomy of the treated limb are the goals of combining radiation with relatively conservative surgery.

In the last decade, wide local excision followed by postoperative radiotherapy delivering approximately 6500 rad in six and a half weeks using a shrinking field technique has yielded local cure rates of 80-90%. Meticulous treatment techniques including immobilization, oblique field arrangements and individualized beam shaping are important to minimize complications. A small strip of soft tissue on the circumference of the extremity must be spared to prevent concentric fibrosis which may cause periperhal edema, joint dysfunction and pain. Treatment portals should include the original tumor site plus a 5-10 cm margin of normal tissue. Field reductions take place at 4500-5000 rad and again at 6000 rad.

Initially, unresectble extremity soft tissue sarcomas can be treated with a course of preoperative radiotherapy delivering 6000 rad over a 6 week period, again with shrinking field techniques. After a suitable rest period of 5-6 weeks, curative preservative surgery can often be undertaken. For bulky lesions, requiring such massive resection that a functionless extremity is produced, amputation remains the best form of management.

Retroperitoneal or thoracic soft tissue sarcomas have a poorer prognosis because complete excision is often not possible. The basic treatment policies outlined for resectable and unresectable extremity lesions still apply. The doses of pre and postoperative irradiation that can safely be delivered are limited by the large volumes that must be treated and the tolerance of normal tissue such as kidney and small intestine. Intraoperative radiotherapy in the form of permanent iodine-125 seed implantation has been of benefit in obtaining local control with improvement survival in patients with residual tumor at surgery. Intraoperative electron beam therapy is also being investigated.

Radiation therapy alone can be considered in patients who are medically inoperable or who refuse surgery. Following high dose irradiation alone of up to 7000 rad, the two-year disease-free survival in such patients is about 15%. Unresectable lesions treated with radiotherapy alone have a local recurrence rate of approximately 60% using conventional fractionation.

Adjuvant Chemotherapy

A prospective randomized study from M.D. Anderson Hospital investigated the use of doxorubicin, vincristine and cyclophosphamide (followed by actinomycin-D after a maximum dose of doxorubicin had been given) in high grade soft tissue sarcomas involving the head and neck, trunk and extremities. No statistically significant difference in disease-free survival was demonstrated in this study. However, a recent report from the National Cancer Institute revealed an improvement in disease-free and overall survival in patients receiving adjuvant chemotherapy with doxorubicin, cyclophosphamide and high-dose methotrexate. This study was a prospective randomized trial with a median follow-up of almost two years. Local therapy consisted of either amputation or wide local resection plus radiotherapy. Local failures occurred in only 2 of 65 patients.

The utility of the AJC staging system for soft tissue sarcomas has been substantiated by the report of the Task Force for Sarcomas and soft tissues, which examined the outcome of 1215 retrospectively staged patients of all histologic subtypes. Five-year survivals by stage are: stage I, 75%; stage II, 55%; stage III, 29%; stage IV, 7%. Overall, the five-year survival rate for soft tissue sarcomas treated by radical surgery or wide local excision plus radiotherapy ranges from 50-60%. The overall incidence of distant metastases is 30-40%. Survival is influenced by the anatomic site of the primary tumor with 69% of patients with extremity lesions surviving five years compared with 33% of patients with trunk lesions. Tumors in a retroperitoneal location fare the worst with only 29% survival at five years. The NCI report of adjuvant chemotherapy in adult soft tissue sarcoma of the extremities yielded a three-year actuarial disease-free survival in 92% of patients receiving chemotherapy compared to 60% in controls.

METASTATIC SOFT TISSUE SARCOMAS

Ten to 15% of patients with soft tissue sarcomas have distant metastases at the time of initial diagnosis. Even in the presence of metastases, local control of the primary tumor may be a problem depending on the metastatic tumor burden and the patient's life expectency. Treatment should proceed in the same fashion as described above with the goal being palliation of local symptomatology. Many soft tissue sarcomas will respond to chemotherapy. Doxorubicin as a single agent yields objective responses in 20-40% of patients. Other active agents include DTIC, cyclophosphamide, vincristine, methotrexate, actinomycin-D and cisplatin. Doxorubicin-based combination chemotherapy regimens result in response rates ranging from 35-40%. Ten percent of patients will have complete responses with 70% of such patients alive for greater than 18 months. Overall, the two-year survival for metastatic soft tissue sarcomas in less than 10%. Some patients with isolated pulmonary metastases can be salvaged by pulmonary wedge resections. Such patients should be carefully selected on the basis of the number of pulmonary metastases (solitary vs multiple), the disease-free interval and the tumor doubling time.

MORBIDITY

Acute

Acute reactions to postoperative radiotherapy are limited to the skin. Postoperative radiotherapy usually does not commence for 2-3 weeks following surgery (when wound healing is complete). Preoperative radiotherapy using doses of 5000-6000 rad has resulted in delayed wound healing.

Chronic

Significant late complications are seen in 6-8% of patients treated with conservative resection and postoperative radiation therapy and include soft tissue necrosis, fracture, constrictive fibrosis, distal lymphedema, nerve and vascular damage, and joint dysfunction. Most of these complications can be avoided or minimized by careful attention to radiotherapeutic techniques. The patient should be instructed to carry out range of motion exercises to maintain mobility by minimizing muscle and tendon shortening. An entire joint is irradiated only when absolutely necessary.

REFERENCES

1. Lindberg RD et al: Conservative surgery and postoperative radiotherapy in 300 adults with soft-tissue sarcomas. Cancer 47:2391-2397, 1981.
2. Rosenberg SA et al: Prospective randomized evaluation of adjuvant chemotherapy in adults with soft tissue sarcomas of the extremities. Cancer 52:424-434, 1983.
3. Tepper J, Rosenberg SA and Glatstein, E: Radiation therapy technique in soft tissue sarcomams of the extremity--policies of treatment at the National Cancer Institute. I J Rad Onc Bio Phys 8:263-273, 1981.
4. Carson JH et al: The place of radiotherapy in the treatment of synovial sarcoma. I J Rad Onc Bio Phys 7:49-53, 1980.
5. Suit HD: Sarcoma of soft tissue. CA 28:284-295, 1978.

Chapter 14

Bone Tumors

BONE SARCOMAS

OVERVIEW

Primary bone malignancies are relatively rare with less than 2500 new cases per year. Multiple myeloma (more correctly a hematologic malignancy) accounts for 40%; osteosarcomas, 28%; chondrosarcomas, 13%; fibrosarcomas arising in bone, 4% and Ewing's sarcoma, 7%.

PATHOLOGY

Osteosarcomas may be subdivided on the basis of their histologic and radiographic characteristics into four subgroups: telangiectatic, central, periosteal and parosteal. Chondrosarcomas have been pathologically classified as dedifferentiated mesenchymal, clear cell and juxtacortical types. Malignant fibrous histiocytoma of bone has also been described. Fibrosarcoma primary in bone histologically resembles soft tissue fibrosarcoma and is thought to arise from the periosteum. Ewing's sarcoma is a round cell tumor of bone involving the medullary cavity and shafts of the long bone as well as ribs, vertebrae and flat bones. Microscopically, it must be differentiated from malignant lymphoma, neuroblastoma and metastatic carcinomas.

CLINICAL FEATURES

Bone sarcomas generally present with pain, often worse at night. There is limb dysfunction, a palpable mass and commonly pathologic fracture. Hematogenous spread, particularly to the lung, is the rule, although there is occasionally also lymph node involvement.

STAGING

A TNM staging system for bone cancer has been suggested by the AJC, but the system has not yet been complete and its usefulness remains to be defined.

WORK-UP

Routine studies include: radiographs of the affected bone, biopsy of the lesion, total body bone scan, angiography, xeroradiographs and CT to detect extension outside the bone. Whole lung tomograms or CT of the chest to rule out lung metastases. For osteosarcoma, serum alkaline phosphatase has shown to be of diagnostic and prognostic significance. The erythrocyte sedimentation rate and white blood cell count correlate with the aggressiveness of Ewing's sarcoma.

TREATMENT AND RESULTS

Osteosarcoma: When these tumors involve extremities, radical amputation is the established treatment. The goal of therapy is to provide a 10 cm margin of apparently normal bone proximal to all scintigraphic and radiographic evidence of tumor. Therefore, some tumors in the distal femur can be treated with a very high above the knee amputation. The local recurrence rate is less than 5%. Osteosarcomas are notoriously radioresistant. Persistent tumor is frequently found in amputation specimens following preoperative doses of 6000 to 6500 rad. Preoperative radiotherapy with doses from 4500 rad to as high as 12,000 rad has failed to improve survival. Postoperative radiotherapy is unneccessary for local control if the above surgical principles are adhered to.

Eighty percent of all patients dying of osteosarcoma have metastatic disease in the lung at autopsy. The use of chemotherapy was instituted to alter this pattern of failure. Combination chemotherapy consisting of vincristine, high dose methotrexate with citrovorum rescue with or without doxorubicin has been employed in several studies, yielding a 60% actuarial disease-free survival compared with a 20% survival for historical controls. The use of historical controls leaves these studies vulnerable to criticism. CT scanning has allowed the identification of patients with definite pulmonary metastases that in the past have gone undetected by other roentgenographic techniques. A recent surgical series reported from the Mayo Clinic where no adjuvant therapy was applied boasts a 40-50% disease-free survival. Furthermore, a recent analysis of prognostic factors in patients at the Karolinska Hospital in Sweden have shown that present day patients have somewhat smaller tumors, which are of a lower grade, indicating that there may be some change in the natural history of this malignancy.

Limb salvage therapy is being investigated and consists of en bloc excision of the primary bone tumor to include 10 cm margins proximal to the tumor as well as wide margins of soft tissue. The skeletal defect is corrected with a prosthetic device or a cadaveric allograft. Surgical management is usually preceded by preoperative chemotherapy, with or without radiotherapy. A two year disease-free survival of 55% with relatively good function in the salvaged limb has been reported.

Adjuvant whole lung irradiation has been attempted using doses of 1500-2000 rad with or wihtout doxorubicin or actinomycin-D. These regimens were not effective in preventing metastases when compared to concurrent controls and yielded results comparable to that of chemotherapy alone. Therefore, this approach is no longer advocated. Once pulmonary metastases develop, surgical resection of even multiple metastases can be considered if the primary tumor is controlled and the lungs are the only site of metastatic spread. This aggressive approach has yielded two-year survivals ranging from 30-60%. If, however, the tumor displays a short doubling time of less than two months, patients are unlikely to benefit from resection. Histology of the primary osteosarcoma correlates with 5-year survival with telangiectatic lesions having a 5% five-year survival; central lesions, 20%; periosteal: 40% and periosteal, 80% five-year survival.

Chondrosarcoma: This second most common primary malignant bone tumor, is managed similar to osteosarcoma with radical surgery being the treatment of choice.

When only local excision is employed, 90% of patients will recur locally. Overall ten-year survival following surgery is approximately 65% and varies according to histologic grade. Eighty-three percent of patients with grade I lesions will live ten years while only 29% of patients with grade III lesions survive at that time.

The experience with radiotherapy as the primary modality for chondrosarcoma is limited. Patients referred for such treatment have unfavorable prognostic factors such as a primary site on the trunk or in the head and neck. Nonetheless complete responses may be obtained in over half of the patients following radical radiotherapy. Since pulmonary metastases are less common with grades I or II chondrosarcomas, the value of chemotherapy is not well established. For metastatic chondrosarcoma, doxorubicin yields a response rate of only 17%. Resection of limited pulmonary metastases may be of benefit.

Fibrosarcoma primary in bone: Radical surgery remains the treatment of choice. The femur, tibia and humerus are commonly involved and are sites amenable to amputation. The prognosis for fibrosarcoma of bone is intermediate between soft tissue fibrosarcomas and osteosarcomas, with a reported five-year survival of about 30%.

Malignant fibrous histiocytoma of bone: Existence of this entity is well established, although the literature is scant on how it should best be managed. Successful management by radical resection and adjuvant chemotherapy has been reported with disease-free intervals ranging from 42-48 months in three patients.

MORBIDITY

Acute

Reactions are related to skin and soft tissue irradiation (See Chapter 3).

Chronic

The late effects of bone irradiation are highly dependent on the patient's age at the time of therapy.

When children are irradiated, radiation-induced bone deformities caused by damage to the growth centers and epiphyseal plate occur. These may be manifested as bone shortening and kyphoscloiosis. Deformity of the skull and facial bones due to growth arrest can also occur. Slipped capital femoral epiphyses is a complication of pelvic irradiation in childhood.

Radiation osteitis is seen as a late effect when adult bone is radiated. Pain may be the presenting symptom. Radiographically, postirradiation osteitis presents as a mixed osteoporotic/sclerotic area that is outlined by the radiation portals. These bones, particularly the pubic rami and femurs, are subject to pathologic fracture. Metastatic disease is the main differential diagnosis and may be excluded by biopsy. When the mandible is affected and bone is exposed due to soft tissue necrosis or ill-advised dental procedures, chronic osteomyelitis and pain are the sequelae.

Radiation-induced sarcoma of bone is another late sequelae of the use of ionizing radiation for the treatment of cancer. Osteosarcomas, fibrosarcomas, chondrosarcomas and malignant fibrous histiocytomas have all been reported. Cahan established criteria to make the diagnosis of radiation-induced sarcomas:

1. Microscopic or radiographic evidence of the initial nonmalignant nature of the involved bone.
2. Sarcomas developing in the area that has been included in radiation portals.
3. Histologic confirmation of the sarcomatous tumor different from the original tumor histology.
4. A significant asymptomatic latent period greater than 5 years from the time of irradiation to the appearance of the sarcoma.

The dose response for tumor induction is not clear. Sarcomas occurring below 1200 rad have been reported; however, the majority occur after doses exceeding 5000 rad. The outlook for radiation-induced sarcomas is essentially the same as spontaneously occurring tumors with an overall survival ranging from 11-28%.

EWING'S SARCOMA

OVERVIEW

Ewing's sarcoma, a small cell malignant tumor of bone, was described in 1921 by James Ewing. Although the tumor is quite radiosensitive, it was almost uniformly lethal due to distant dissemination. Early series reported five-year survivals ranging from 4-10% whether the primary tumor was managed with surgery or with radiotherapy. Ewing's sarcoma is discussed separately from the other bone sarcomas because its current management represents a paradigm for multidisciplinary treatment, which has resulted in greatly improved cure rates.

PATHOLOGY

These anaplastic tumors consist of sheets of round, oval or spindle-shaped cells with prominent nuclei and frequently pronouced necrosis. This histologic pattern makes it difficult to distinguish this tumor from undifferentiated carcinoma, neuroblastoma or high grade lymphoma. However, non-cleft nuclear margins are a distinguishing feature from the lymphomas. PAS positivity may be used to help differentiated Ewing's sarcoma from neuroblastoma.

CLINICAL FEATURES

Ewing's sarcoma occurs most commonly in young adults during the second decade of life, with a peak incidence ranging from 12-16 years. The male:female ratio is 3:2. Localized pain is the most common presenting feature. The diaphysis of the femur is commonly involved, although the tumor can arise in any bone. X-ray shows a diffuse lytic process often with a soft tissue mass growing out from the bone producing periosteal elevation with a characteristic "onion skin" appearance. Fever and leukocytosis are frequent. When the tumor arises in the pelvis, patients can present with voiding difficulty secondary to sacral plexus dysfunction, which results in a neurogenic bladder. Brain metastases have recently been recognized as a site for relapse.

WORK-UP

The diagnostic work-up is almost identical to that described for other bone sarcomas but should include biopsy of the primary tumor. These tumors may be necrotic and secondarily infected and resemble osteomyelitis grossly. Ewing's sarcoma metastasizes to the lungs but also comonly involves the skeleton, making a bone scan mandatory. A CT scan is helpful to evaluate the extraosseous extension of the local bone tumor. If vertebral involvement is present, myelography is indicated. Bone marrow biopsy to rule out subclinical disease is essential. Anemia, elevation of the sedimentation rate and elevated LDH carry a poor prognosis.

TREATMENT AND RESULTS

Ewing's sarcoma is a systemic disease from the outset. Multimodality therapy consists of local treatment of the primary tumor and intensive combination chemotherapy for occult or overt metastatic disease. Radiotherapy to the primary site provides adequate local control with preservation of function. Doses in the range of 4500-6500 rad in 5-6 weeks provides a local control rate of about 75% and when combined with chemotherapy the control rate approaches 90%. Radiotherapeutic treatment involves inclusion of the entire bone since the primary may extend far beyond the radiographically involved portion of the bone, infiltrating along the periosteum and into the adjacent soft tissue. After a dose of 4500 rad, a shrinking field technique is employed to boost the primary for an additional 1000-1500 rad. When an extremity is treated, a soft tissue tunnel is spared to preserve function. The role of surgery is often limited to establishing a diagosis by incisional biopsy or excision of "expendable bones" such as ribs or the scapula. Local control of bulky tumors in the pelvic bones is suboptimal with radiation and chemotherapy. Surgical debulking of pelvic tumors is being investigated.

Adjuvant chemotherapy incorporating 3 or 4 cytotoxic agents (cyclophosphamide, actinomycin-D, vincristine and doxorubicin) has yielded four-year actuarial disease-free survivals of 70-80%. These same agents have a 60% response rate when used to treat metastatic disease. Adjuvant radiotherapy has been used prophylactically for the prevention of cerebral and pulmonary metastases. Total body irradiation was also attempted as one of the earliest forms of systemic management, but has been supplanted by the advent of effective chemotherapy.

MORBIDITY

The combined use of radiotherapy and combination chemotherapy, particularly adriamycin, may be associated with significant toxicity. Children below age five may develop severely compromised function of extremities secondary to postirradiation fibrosis. Attention has recently been focused on the development of second malignancies in long-term survivors of Ewing's sarcoma. To date these have been secondary osteosarcomoas and fibrosarcomas and may be related to radiation doses to the bone greater than 5000 rad.

PRIMARY LYMPHOMA IN BONE

These tumors arise from lymphoid elements in the marrow cavity and may be subclassified according to major histologic types with emphasis on nuclear morphology: cleaved, non-cleaved and pleomorphic. The pathology is often that of a diffuse histiocytic tumor, although diffuse poorly differentiated lymphocytic and lymphoblastic tumors do occur. Formerly, the histiocytic variety was known as primary reticulum cell sarcoma of bone.

Similar to Ewing's sarcoma, the pathologic extent of the tumor is usually underestimated by radiographic studies. Node metastases have been reported in 20% of patients in one series. The average age of patients with this disease is 35. Pain is again the presenting symptom.

The work-up for primary lymphoma in bone is similar to other presentations of non-Hodgkin's lymphoma. A lymphangiogram is highly desirable. Bone marrow involvement should be ruled out by bilateral iliac crest biopsies. A bone scan may reveal multiple sites of involvement.

Primary lymphoma of bone is radiosensitive and local control can be achieved in 80-90% of patients with modern radiotherapeutic techniques. Portals should include the entire bone as well as periosteal soft tissue masses. A dose of 4000 rad in four weeks is delivered to this field, and shrinking field techniques are utilized to deliver an additional 1000 rad to the primary tumor site. Regional lymph nodes are included only if they are immediately adjacent to the treatment area or if clinically involved. This regimen yields a five-year survival of 60% with a 50% disease-free surival. The role of adjuvant chemotherapy requires further study.

REFERENCES

1. Mankin HJ: Advances in diagnosis and treatment of bone tumors. N Eng J Med 300:543-545, 1979.
2. Chabner BA et al (ed): Cancer Treatment Reports, vol 62, pp 187-313. U.S. Department of Health, Education and Welfare, Washington, D.C., 1978.
3. Brostrom, L et al: Can historical controls be used in current clinical trials in osteosarcoma? analysis of prognostic factors: I J Rad Onc Bio Phys 6:1711-1715, 1980.
4. Weisenburger TH et al: Multidisiciplinary "limb salvage" treatment of soft tissue and skeletal sarcomas: I J Rad Onc Bio Phys 7:1495-1499, 1981.
5. Dosoretz DE et al: Radiation therapy for primary lymphoma of bone. Cancer 51:44-46, 1983.
6. Smith J: Radiation-induced sarcoma of bone: clinical and radiographic findings in 43 patients irradiated for soft tissue neoplasms. Clinical Radiology 33:205-221, 1982.

Chapter 15

Childhood Tumors

OVERVIEW

Cancer is the second most common cause of death in children in the United States. In the last two decades great strides have been made toward curing many childhood cancers through multidisciplinary management. Unique to the treatment of pediatric neoplasia is the fact that the patient's normal tissues are in phases of development and growth which render them quite susceptible to damage from chemotherapy and radiotherapy. In addition, the patient is quite vulnerable to psychological trauma from aggressive antineoplastic management, which often isolates the patient from family and friends.

The goal of treatment is the same as in the adult patient; namely, uncomplicated cure. However, because of the sensitivity of the child's developing tissues to toxic side effects, this is not easily attained. When the child is cured of his malignant disease, the longer life expectancy makes him more likely to manifest late side effects of treatment. The challenge to pediatric oncologists and radiotherapists in the coming years will be to minimize treatment complications without sacrificing the impressive gains in survival and tumor control achieved to date.

This chapter will discuss the clinical characteristics and management of Wilms' tumor, neuroblastoma and rhabdomyosarcoma which collectively account for 20% of pediatric malignancies. Discussion of these three tumors will serve to illustrate the triumphs that can be obtained using a combined-modality approach as well as the attendant morbidity in the pediatric age group. Leukemias and lymphomas account for 40-45% of malignancies in children under 15 years of age. The radiotherapeutic aspects of their management are outlined in Chapter 8. CNS tumors, including medullobastoma, account for 20% of all childhood malignant tumors and are discussed in Chapter 5.

Osteogenic sarcoma and Ewing's sarcoma make up 4% of childhood cancers, and their treatment is discussed in Chapter 14. Management of retinoblastoma, another rare pediactric malignancy, is detailed in Chapter 6.

WILMS' TUMOR

PATHOLOGY

Wilms' tumor or nephroblastoma arises in the renal parenchyma and produces deformity of the pyelocalyceal system. Microscopically, it is an embryonic tumor made up of very immature renal parenchymal (blastemic) cells with varying degrees of epithelial and mesenchymal differentiation. Unfavorable histologic features, which correlate with a poor prognosis, have been identified: focal and diffuse anaplasia, "rhabdoid" sarcoma and clear cell sarcoma. The rhabdoid variant is associated with intracranial neoplasms, while the clear cell sarcoma variant has a tendency to metastasize to bone.

CLINICAL FEATURES

Wilms' tumor is the most common intra-abdominal tumor of childhood with the median age at diagnosis of approximately 3.5 years and 75% occurring before age 5. Congenital abnormalities of the urogenital tract, hemihypertrophy and aniridia are commonly associated with Wilms' tumor. The usual presentation is that of asymptomatic abdominal distention or a palpable upper abdominal mass. The tumor may also present with abdominal pain, fever, hematuria or malaise. Hypertension and renal failure are uncommon. Bilateral renal involvement will be present in 5-10% of cases. There is a slight male preponderance.

STAGING

A clinicopathologic staging system has evolved from the grouping system used by the National Wilms' Tumor Study (NWTS).

Stage I	Tumor limited to the kidney and completely excised
Stage II	Tumor extends beyond the kidney, but is completely excised

Stage III	Residual nonhematogenous tumor confined to the abdomen
Stage IV	Hematogenous metastases
Stage V	Bilateral renal involvement at diagnosis

WORK-UP

Intravenous pyelography is the single most useful study in the differential diagnosis of a large abdominal mass and will lead to the correct diagnosis in 95% of cases. IVP will show a parenchymal kidney lesion destorting the calyceal system and will usually differentiate the mass lesion from other disorders such as splenomegaly, neuroblastoma, hydronephrosis, renal carbuncle, benign teratoma, cystic kidney disease and lymphoma. CT scanning, ultrasound and arteriography may also be useful. Metastatic work-up should include chest radiographs, liver/spleen and bone scans which may be done in the preoperative or postoperative period.

TREATMENT

Surgery

Nephrectomy is indispensible to the curative management of patients with Wilms' tumor. A large transverse abdominal incision is employed which allows exploration of the entire abdomen with particular attention to the contralateral kidney which may be involved in 5-10% of cases. Sampling of suspicious regional lymph nodes should be carried out. Radical lymphadenectomy is no longer advocated. Every effort should be made to avoid spillage of tumor.

Radiation Therapy

Treatment concepts have evolved as a result of the first two intergroup National Wilms' Tumor Studies as well as trials organized by the International Society of Pediatric Oncology. Routine postoperative radiotherapy has been shown to be unnecessary in patients with stage I disease with favorable histology. These patients do receive adjuvant actinomycin-D and vincristine. The present (third) National Wilms' Tumor Study is investigating the role of postoperative radiation in stage II disease randomizing these patients to receive 2000 rad postoperatively or no radiotherapy. Stage III patients will be randomized to receive either 1000 rad or 2000 rad postoperatively. The volume of tissue irradiated in these patients includes the tumor bed as defined by the preoperative IVP. The fields traditionally encompass the entire vertebral bodies to minimize the kyphoscoliosis that may be produced. The current NWTS policy for patients with unfavorable histology is to deliver postoperative radiotherapy to the tumor bed in all patients because of the high frequency of local recurrence.

Chemotherapy

Actinomycin-D, vincristine and doxorubicin are extremely effective in the treatment of Wilms' tumor. The combination of actinomycin-D and vincristine proved to be effective in reducing both local and distant disease in the treatment of stage I patients. Six months of therapy has been shown to be as effective as 15 months. The third National Wilms' Tumor Study is exploring the optimal combination of actinomycin-D, vincristine and doxorubicin in the more advanced stages of the disease. Intensifications of the treatment regimens for unfavorable histologic subtypes is also being investigated.

RESULTS

The four-year disease-free survival of patients with stage I disease approaches 90% in patients less than two years of age and varies from 57-76% in patients greater than or equal to two years of age at diagnosis. The four-year relapse-free survival in stage II or III disease ranges from 57-79%.

Pulmonary metastases may successfully be managed with combined-modality therapy. Bilateral lung irradiation to 1200-1400 rad is given with concomitant chemotherapy. If pulmonary metastases fail to respond or recur following irradiation, surgical resection of pulmonary nodules can be curative. The cure rate for patients with stage IV disease approaches 60%.

MORBIDITY

Acute

Gastrointestinal toxicity (nausea, vomiting, diarrhea) is an acute toxic effect of combined modality treatment with chemotherapy and radiation. Because actinomycin-D and doxorubicin are radiosensitizers, increased skin reactions can be observed. Radiation hepatitis can occur.

Chronic

Skeletal growth retardation can be seen resulting in kyphoscoliosis. This can be minimized by extending the radiation portals across the midline to include both epiphyseal growth centers of the vertebral bodies. This portal should extend across the midline far enough to allow irradiation of the entire para-aortic lymph node chain, yet spare the healthy contralateral kidney. Therefore, radiation nephritis is generally not a problem except in the case of bilateral renal involvement where is is necessary to irradiate a portion of the contralateral kidney. Atrophy of the trunk musculature and skin changes are also seen as late effects. These soft tissue effects may contribute to the development of scoliosis.

Other possible late toxic effects of combined-modality treatment include radiation pneumonitis and cardiomyopathy (doxorubicin related). Second malignant neoplasms are also being recognized in long-term survivors. Bone sarcomas are the most frequent second tumors reported and often arise in radiation portals. Genetic predisposition of the development of malignancy is likely an important factor.

NEUROBLASTOMA

PATHOLOGY

Neuroblastoma is a malignant tumor of the sympathetic ganglion tissue. Microscopically, the tumor cells are small, round, neuroblasts with hyperchromatic nuclei with a tendency to form "pseudo-rosettes" about central primitive nerve fibers. Varying degrees of differentiation will be present in the same tumors with some tumors spontaneously maturing into ganglioneuromas. Elements of neuroblastoma may be found in the adrenal glands of 0.5% of newborns. The cell of origin is believed to be the neural crest stem cell. Often these tumors are biochemically active, producing catecholamines and their metabolites in 75% of patients.

CLINICAL FEATURES

Neuroblastoma is the second commonest solid tumor in children, accounting for 7% of the total cases of childhood cancer. The median age at diagnosis is two years with neuroblastoma being the most frequently diagnosed tumor in the neonatal period. The clinical presentation depends on the site of the primary tumor and the presence of distant metastases. Sixty percent of patients have intra-abdominal primary sites, either in the adrenal gland (40%) or the paraspinal sympathetic ganglia (20%). The mediastinal ganglia are the site of origin in another 15%. Infants may present with abdominal extension secondary to local tumor growth or hepatic metastases. Jaundice, ascites, malaise, lethargy, subcutaneous nodules, proptosis, orbital ecchymoses, opsoclonus, anorexia, diarrhea, weight loss, Horner's syndrome and spinal cord compression may be other signs and symptoms of the disease. These patients generally appear "sick", in contrast to patients with Wilms' tumor.

STAGING

Staging is based on primary tumor size as well as the extent and sites of dissemination. According to the staging system proposed by Evans et al, 9% of patients have stage I; 14%, stage II; 11%, stage III; 11%, stage IV-S and 55%, stage IV. Staging does correlate with prognosis. Other factors of strong prognostic importance not included in the staging system are age and primary site. In children under 1 year of age, the 2-year disease-free survival rate is 75%, while for children older than 2-years, only 12% are disease free at 2 years. The outcome for primary cervical or thoracic tumors is more favorable than abdominal presentations.

Clinical Stage of Neuroblastoma in Children

I	Tumor confined to organ or structure of origin.
II	Tumor extending in continuity beyond organ or structure of origin but not crossing midline. Regional lymph nodes on the homolateral side may be involved
III	Tumor extending in continuity beyond the midline. Regional lymph nodes may be involved bilaterally.
IV	Remote disease involving, skelton, organs, soft tissue, or distant lymph node groups
IV-S	Patients usually younger than age 1 and would otherwise be classified as having stage I or II but have remote disease confined to one or more of the following sites: liver, skin, or bone marrow (without radiographic evidence of bone metastases)

WORK-UP

In all children suspected of harboring neuroblastoma, the following studies should be performed: radiographs of the abdomen and chest, IVP, bone scan, skeletal survey, liver/spleen scan, assays for urinary catecholamine metabolites (VMA, HVA, cystathionine and beta-aminoisobutyric acid), bone marrow aspiration and biopsy, abdominal ultrasound and abdominal CT scan. When neuroblastoma presents as an adrenal tumor, it may be calcified, displacing the kidney downward on IVP. An intrathoracic neuroblastoma is most often located in the posterior mediastinum and may invade the intravertebral foramina creating a "dumbbell" tumor which may cause spinal cord compression. In such cases, selected radiographs and myelography are required. Depending on the presenting stage, the tissue diagnosis can be established by biopsy of lymph nodes, subcutaneous nodules or bone marrow. Otherwise, the diagnosis is established at exploratory laparotomy or thoracotomy.

TREATMENT AND RESULTS

Surgery

When neuroblastoma is localized, surgical resection is the treatment of choice. Surgery need not be "radical", although nephrectomy is advocated for adrenal tumors. If excision has been complete, no adjuvant therapy is required. "Second-look" surgery may have a role in the management of initially inoperable stage III tumors, which have been debulked by radiation therapy and chemotherapy. The relapse-free survival at 2 years for patients with stage I and stage II disease approximates 90%.

Radiation Therapy

The role of radiotherapy in the management of neuroblastoma is either as a surgical adjuvant or for palliation.

Postoperative doses of 1500-3500 rad for residual microscopic or gross tumor have been employed with good local control. Doses in the range of 1000-2000 rad are quite effective for palliation of bone pain, hepatomegaly, neurologic symptoms and other manifestations of metastatic disease. Radiotherapy may also serve to debulk primary tumors in advanced stage neuroblastoma for subsequent resection at a "second-look" operation. Fractionated total body irradiation has been attempted in disseminated neuroblastoma without success.

Chemotherapy

Approximately two-thirds of patients present with widely disseminated neuroblastoma, making chemotherapy the mainstay of management. Active agents include cyclophosphamide, melphelan, doxorubicin, DTIC, VM-26 and cisplatin. When used in combination, complete responses can be obtained in 30-40% of stage IV patients with another 30% obtaining partial responses. These responses tend to be short-lived and the 2-year disease-free survival in such patients is less than 10%. Chemotherapy has not been helpful in reducing the recurrence or metastatic rate in early stage neuroblastoma. Its role as adjuvant therapy in stage III disease remains to be defined. Because of the unsatisfactory results to date, the chemotherapeutic management of stage IV disease remains investigational. High dose chemotherapy with or without total body irradiation with autologous bone marrow rescue is being investgated in some centers. Monoclonal antibodies and retinoic acid are presently undergoing preclinical investigations and may have a future role in therapy.

Children with stage IV-S neuroblastoma often undergo spontaneous remissions and enjoy 80% survival. Treatment is usually withheld unless the patient develops symptoms related to tumor bulk. Low dose irradiation and/or low dose cyclophosphamide or vincristine will result in sufficient tumor regression to relieve mechanical symptoms due to tumor bulk. The primary tumor should be resected.

MORBIDITY

The sequelae of combined-modality treatment for neuroblastoma are similar to those of Wilms' tumor patients.

RHABDOMYOSARCOMA

OVERVIEW

Rhabdomyosarcoma is the most common soft tissue sarcoma of childhood representing the third most common solid tumor and the seventh leading cause of cancer death. An interdisciplinary approach using surgery, radiation and multiagent chemotherapy has been pioneered by the Intergroup Rhabdomyosarcoma Study and has led to a tripling of the two-year survival rate for this tumor in the last 20 years.

PATHOLOGY

Rhabdomyosarcomas are derived from embryonic mesenchymal cells. Three distinct variants are described. The *pleomorphic* variety is that seen primarily in adults and consists of spindle and "strap" cells and will not be further discussed in this chapter. The *alveolar* subtype is comprised of round cells with reticulin-staining trabeculae and is often found in adolescents and young adults. The embryonal variant is most commonly found in children. Microscopically, it consists of spindle shaped, round and "tadpole" or "raquet" cells, often with a myxomatous matrix. A botryoid subtype of embryonal carcinoma is so named because of its gross appearance as "a bunch of grapes" often growing into a hollow viscus. These polypoid growths are soft, glistening and grow in clusters. Sarcoma botryoides is found in the bladder, prostate and vagina of infants.

CLINICAL FEATURES

The peak incidence of this disease is between the ages of 2 and 5, with 70% of patients occurring before age 10. The male to female ratio is approximately 1.4:1. The anatomic sites of origin are the head and neck regions (35%), extremities (25%), GU tract (20%), trunk (10%), retroperitoneum (5%) and other sites (5%). Signs and symptoms are related to the development of mass lesions at the various anatomic sites.

STAGING

The Intergroup Rhabdomyosarcoma Study grouping is most commonly employed.

Stage I	Localized disease, completely resected
Stage IA	Confined to the muscle or organ of origin
Stage IB	Contiguous involvement with infiltration outside the muscle or organ of origin with microscopic confirmation of complete resection and no lymph node involvement
Stage II	Localized disease, microscopic residua
Stage IIA	Grossly resected but with residual microscopic disease and no lymph node involvement
Stage IIB	Regional nodal disease completely resected with no microscopic residua
Stage IIC	Regional nodal involvement, grossly resected but with evidence of microscopic residua

Stage III Incomplete resection or biopsy with gross residual regional disease
Stage IV Distant metastases at time of diagnosis

WORK-UP

Because of the propensity of rhabdomyosarcoma to spread via lymphactics and hematogenously, clinical assessment of regional lymph nodes is manditory. Lymphangiography for lower extremity and GU lesions may be helpful. Chest radiographs and conventional or computed whole lung tomography are required to rule out pulmonary metastases. A CT scan is also useful in the evaluation of pelvic and other primary sites. Liver/spleen scan, bone scan and bone marrow aspiration are routine.

TREATMENT AND RESULTS

Surgery

Formerly, radical surgery was the treatment of choice but with the advent of effective chemotherapy, more limited surgical tumor excision with preservation of the involved organ is preferred. Since there is a better outlook when there is no gross residual tumor, total excision is preferred over simple biopsy. Because of anatomic considerations in the head and neck region, it is often difficult to perform wide excision of tumor with "an envelope of normal tissue" and biopsy may be the only feasible procedure. For orbital primaries, biopsy alone followed by adjuvant treatment is preferred over exenteration. The high incidence of lymph node involvement makes elective nodal dissections for GU, head and neck, pelvic and extremity lesions reasonable. Tumors tend to extend along facial planes for considerable distances. Surgery alone is rarely curative because of distant spread and local recurrence.

Radiation Therapy

Relatively high doses of radiation (5000-6000 rad in 5-6 weeks) are required to control rhabdomyosarcoma. The use of doses less than 4000 rad have resulted in an unacceptable incidence of local failure despite adjuvant chemotherapy. Usually generous volumes of the involved muscle compartment must be encompassed in the treatment portals. The inclusion of regional lymph nodes is neither necessary nor desirable. Treatment techniques vary with the anatomic site treated. For stage I patients, postoperative tumor bed irradiation does not improve local control or that obtained with adjuvant chemotherapy alone. For stage III and IV patients, VAC plus doxorubicin is commonly utilized and radiation therapy to the primary site and metastatic deposits is given six weeks postoperatively. Techniques and dose are related to anatomic site and amount of residual tumor. Orbital and nasopharyngeal tumors should be treated to doses to 5000-6000 rad following biopsy alone. At other sites, if wide excision yields margins negative for tumor, no postoperative radiotherapy is indicated. When microscopic disease is present, a postoperative dose of 3000-4000 rad is given.

The prognosis is related to initial stage. The five-year disease-free survival for stage I patients is approximately 80% and for stage II, 75%. At two years, 75% of patients with stage III disease will be alive and 35% of patients with stage IV disease survive.

Chemotherapy

Chemotherapy is essential in the management of rhabdomyosarcoma. Active agents include actinomycin-D, vincristine, cyclosphosphamide doxorubicin, DTIC, bleomycin, cisplatin, BCNU and methotrexate. The combination of vincristine, actinomycin-D and cytoxan (VAC) is administered to stage I and II patients.

MORBIDITY

The sequelae of treatment are qualitatively similar to those seen in Wilms' tumor patients but quantitatively may be more pronouced because of the higher radiation dose usually required to control local disease. For head and neck tumors, facial deformities related to growth retardation of facial bones is seen.

REFERENCES

1. Maurer HM: Current concepts in cancer: solid tumors in children. New Eng J Med 299:1345-1348, 1978.

2. Cohen MD: A rational approach to the radiologic evaluation of children with Wilms' tumor. Cancer 50:887-892, 1982.
3. Belasco J, D'Angio GJ: Wilms' tumor. CA 31:258-270, 1981.
4. D'Angio GJ et al: The treatment of Wilms' tumor: results of the second national Wilms' tumor study: Cancer 47:2302-2311, 1981.
5. Seeger RC et al: Neuroblastoma: clinical perspectives, monoclonal antibodies, and retinoic acid. Ann Int Med 92:873-884, 1982.
6. Evans AE et al: Do infants with stage IV-S neuroblastoma need treatment? Arch Dis Child 56:271-274, 1981.
7. Maurer HM et al: The Intergroup Rhabdomyosarcoma Study: Update, November 1978. J Natl Cancer Inst (Monograph) 56:61-68, 1981.
8. Raney RB, Jr et al: Prognosis of children with soft tissue sarcoma who relapse after achieving a complete response: a report from the Intergroup Rhabdomyosarcoma Study I. Cancer 52:44-50, 1983.
9. Sutow WW, Vietti TJ and Fernbach DJ (ed): Clinical Pediactrics Oncology, 3rd edition, C.V. Morley, St. Louis, 1984.
10. Schweisguth O: Solid Tumors in Children, John Wiley & Sons, New York, 1982.

Chapter 16

Radiotherapeutic Emergencies

OVERVIEW

Problems arising from tumor infiltration of the central nervous system (CNS) or mediastinum may require relatively rapid radiotherapeutic intervention. Manifestations of CNS involvement requiring radiotherapy to halt progressive neurologic compromise include spinal cord compression, meningeal tumor infiltration, and brain metastases. Symptoms of superior vena cava obstruction and airway compression due to malignancies involving the mediastinum can also be effectively diminished or reversed by radiotherapy.

The necessity for rapid treatment is determined by the severity of the clinical problem and its rate of onset and progression. In most circumstances, the treatment is most efficacious when administered when the patient has minimal symptoms. However, apart from the treatment of spinal cord compression and occasionally superior vena cava syndrome, true radiotherapeutic emergencies (where therapy is required within several hours of the diagnosis) are relatively uncommon. Management of brain metastases or meningeal infiltration are rarely if ever radiotherapeutic emergencies and are dealt with in Chapter 17 on palliation.

SPINAL CORD COMPRESSION

OVERVIEW

Over 95% of spinal cord compressions are due to extramedullary malignancy. Intramedullary metastases or primary spinal cord malignancies (gliomas, ependymomas and hemangiomas) are rare. Tumors that arise in or metastasize to bone can cause spinal cord compression by invasion of the epidural space.

PATHOLOGY

Lung, breast, prostate and renal cell carcinoma comprise over 90% of malignancies which may give rise to cord compression. Lymphoma, myeloma and sarcoma may also cause extradural spinal cord compression.

CLINICAL FEATURES

The clinical presentation of cord compression can be divided into the prodromal and compressive phases. The prodromal phase is characterized by local pain, radicular pain and local tenderness. The compressive phase includes weakness, sensory deficits and autonomic dysfunction. Weakness usually precedes sensory loss, but occasionally they may develop together. Autonomic dysfunction may occur early and may manifest as hesitancy and urgency. Loss of sphincter control and paraplegia develop late in the compressive phase.

WORK-UP

History and physical examination with careful neurologic assessment. Knowledge of sensory dermatome distribution is key in clinically determing the level of compression. (See Figure 16.1)

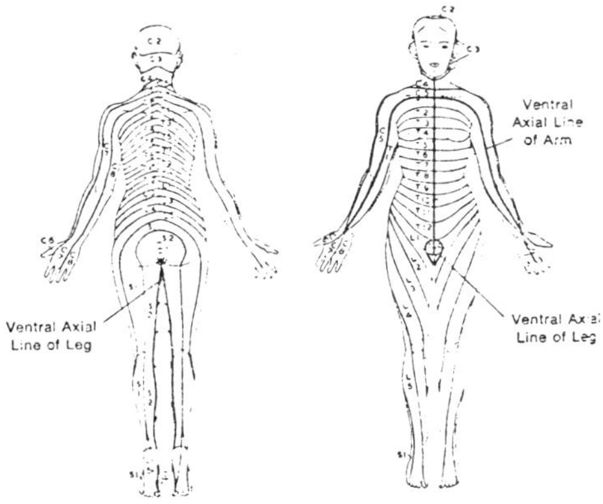

Figure 16.1. Dermatome sensory chart. (from Keegan)

Radiographs of the spine show bony abnormalities at the suspected level of compression in over two-thirds of patients. A myelogram is essential to establish the exact location and extent of compression. The extent of compression is usually limited to the region between one or two vertebral bodies. The upper limits of a complete block should be documented by cisternal puncture if clinically indicated. Multiple sites of spinal cord metastases may be seen in 20% of patients. CSF fluid should be obtained at the time of myelogram and evaluated without delay for cytology, cell count, protein and glucose. CT scan with metrizamide contrast may be useful in evaluating suspected cases of spinal cord compression with negative myelograms.

TREATMENT

A multidisciplinary approach is required in the management of spinal cord compression. After the diagnosis has been made clinically, corticosteroids should be administered. Presently, high doses of dexamethasone (16-100 mg/day) are recommended with rapid tapering as tolerated. Surgical intervention with a decompressive laminectomy is indicated when (1) a histologic diagnosis of the primary malignancy has not been established, (2) progression occurs during irradiation, or (3) a relapse occurs within the irradiated field and spinal cord tolerance has been reached or would be exceeded by further radiation. Operative mortality is low (< 5%); however, significant morbidity may result in 10-33% of patients. Since complete removal of tumor is virtually impossible and postoperative radiation improves prognosis, prevents tumor growth and relieves pain, all surgically decompressed patients should receive postoperative radiation.

It previously was held that radiation therapy alone, without initial decompressive laminectomy was appropriate only in those patients with slowly progressive neurologic symptoms, incomplete block or epidural metastases below the level of the conus medullaris. However, it is doubtful whether initial surgery offers improved prognosis over radiation alone, even with rapidly progressive neurologic deficits or complete block. Also, it is not clear whether patients with known relatively radioresistant tumors benefit from surgical decompression over radiation alone, since treatment results are poor with such tumors regardless of treatment chosen. Radiation therapy is therefore the treatment of choice for most patients with spinal cord compression. The radiation treatment fractionation schedule chosen may vary with tumor type, rate of onset and progression of cord compression, and physician preference. Suitable doses range from 3000 rad to 4000 rad over 2-4 weeks. Treatment should be initiated within a few hours after documentation of a block on myelogram.

RESULTS

Treatment outcome is dependent on three major factors. (1) Severity of pretreatment dysfunction, (2) rapidity of onset, and (3) histology. Other factors of lesser importance in prognosis include location (e.g. lower thoracic spine better than upper), presence of bony abnormalities (worse in presence) and duration of pretreatment dysfunction (worse with increasing duration).

(1) Patients with severe dysfunction prior to initiation of treatment have little chance of significant improvement, thus underscoring the importance of early diagnosis. Less than 10% of patients with paraplegia at diagnosis become ambulatory. Similarly, patients with loss of sphincter control seldom regain function. However, 35% of patients paraparetic before treatment remain ambulatory post-treatment. The duration of improvement is similar for both surgery and radiation versus radiation alone with 75% of those ambulatory following radiation remaining ambulatory at 6 months or longer, and 50% remaining ambulatory at 12 months or longer (in patients surviving that long).

(2) Slowly progressive neurologic symptoms are associated with a better prognosis than are rapidly progressing deficits. Additionally, the more rapidly the compression develops the shorter the time one has to relieve compression before the effects of compression are irreversible. However, when paresis or paralysis develops in less than 48 hours, surgical decompression

is probably no better than radiotherapy (as mentioned, controversy exists regarding treatment of rapidly progressive tumors).

(3) Histologically, the lymphomas and myelomas are associated with a better prognosis than carcinomas. If one measures a satisfactory result by the ability to control sphincters and ambulate unassisted for three months or longer postradiation, then approximately 50% of patients with lymphoma or myeloma will have a satifactory result. This compares to approximately 33% with breast or prostate primaries and only 10% with lung or kidney primaries.

MORBIDITY

For radiation effects on spinal cord see Chapter 5.

SUPERIOR VENA CAVA OBSTRUCTION

OVERVIEW

Obstruction of the superior vena cava from a mediastinal malignancy produces a clinical syndrome of acute or subacute onset that is often relieved with prompt radiotherapy.

PATHOLOGY

In 75% of patients, obstruction is due to lung cancer. About 5% of patients with cancer of the lung develop superior vena cava syndrome. Oat cell carcinoma is the most frequent histologic type. Malignant lymphoma (usually diffuse NH lymphoma) and metastatic cancer to the mediastinum may also occasionally give rise to the syndrome. Benign causes such as goiter, aortic aneurism and fibrosing mediastinum are rare.

CLINICAL FEATURES & WORK-UP

Obstruction of venous drainage in the upper thorax results in facial edema, plethora, conjunctival edema, and distention of veins of the neck and thorax in the majority of patients. Tachypnea, cyanosis, and upper extremity edema are also seen.

The clinical picture is often striking and extensive diagnostic testing is usually not warranted. If the tumor type is not already known, establishment of histology by sputum cytology, bronchoscopy with biopsy or SC nodal biopsy should be attempted if the clinical condition permits. Initiation of treatment should not be unnecessarily delayed. Location of the tumor is usually adequately determined by chest x-ray alone. Occasionally, radioisotopic scans aid in determination of the area and extent of obstruction. Superior vena cavagrams are not required in most instances.

TREATMENT

Radiotherapy is the most important modality in the treatment of SVC obstruction. Initial treatment usually consists of several high dose fractions (300 to 400 rad) daily for the first 3 days. This is followed buy conventional (180 to 200 rad) daily treatment to a total dose which depends on histology and clinical setting. Lymphomas are generally treated to 3000 to 4000 rad, while carcinomas require 4000 to 5000 rad or more to achieve significant term local control. Lower doses are used when disease is widespread and short term palliation is the only goal.

Chemotherapy in addition to radiotherapy adds nothing to local palliation over radiotherapy alone in most malignancies. However, chemotherapy has been used successfully as the primary treatment of patients with SVC obstruction due to oat cell carcinoma and occasionally other chemoresponive tumors such as germ cell tumors. It provides effective palliation in most patients and additionally affords systemic management. Radiotherapy may be required in those patients with oat cell carcinoma who have large or rapidly progressive disease.

Additional treatments include:

1. Diuretics - Furosemide (20-80 mg daily in divided doses) is often used during the initial several days of treatment to relieve edema. Watch for hyponatremia and hypokalemia.

2. Steroids - May be of value, particularly when respiratory compromise is present.

3. Anticoagulants - May be of value, particularly if SVC does not respond to radiotherapy since thrombosis may be present. (Here a superior vena cavagram or radionuclide vena cavagram may be useful to determine whether thrombotic obstruction is present).

RESULTS

There is usually good, prompt symptomatic relief within 3-4 days of initiation of radiation; three-fourths of patients have relief of symptoms by 3-4 days and over 90% by one week. Objective signs of response to treatment are seen somewhat later. Two-thirds of patients have objective response by 7 days and 90% within 2 weeks of treatment initiation. Patients without response to radiation may have thrombosis and anticoagulants should be considered. Overall survival is poor, since most patients with SVC have lung cancer, but 45% of patients with lymphoma will survive over 2 years.

AIRWAY COMPRESSION

OVERVIEW

Carcinoma of the lung, trachea and esophagus may give rise to compression of the trachea or carina. Hemoptysis, dyspnea and stridor may result. Surgical resection, cryotherapy and laser treatment are possible management techniques. Radiotherapy is often indicated for incompletely resected lesions or for compression due to extrinsic masses. Corticosteroids are given prior to radiation. Daily radiation is given at 200 rad doses to total doses of 5000 rad or more. Palliation may be obtained but long term survival is rare.

REFERENCES

1. Bruckman J and Bloomer W: Management of spinal cord compression. Semin Oncol 5:1978.
2. Perez CA, Presant CA and Amburg AL: Management of superior vena cava syndrome. Semin Oncol 5:123-134, 1978.

Chapter 17

Palliation

OVERVIEW

Depending on anatomic location, the unchecked growth of primary or metastatic malignancies can cause a number of distressing symptoms such as hemorrhage, bone pain, visceral pain, seizure, paralysis and asphyxia. The role of radiotherapy for the relief of these symptoms is well established. Despite the fact that perhaps half of all radiation treatments are given with palliative intent, this aspect of the field receives little discussion in major textbooks of radiation therapy. This chapter deals with the more common problems presenting for palliative management, such as bone, brain and liver metastases. The role of radiotherapy in the management of metastatic non-squamous cancer of unknown origin is also discussed here. Less common entities such as choroidal metastases are dealt within the chapters discussing the appropriate organ systems. The management of superior vena cava syndrome and spinal cord compression is detailed in Chapter 16.

Palliative treatment must be individualized taking into consideration such varibles as performance status, extent of disease, life expectancy, previous treatment, patient convenience and expense. It makes little sense to deliver a five week palliative course of radiotherapy if the patient has a life expectancy of only three months. On the other hand, the same course of treatment may be reasonable for an ambulatory patient with breast cancer whose only clinical site of disease is bone. Such a patient could live for many years so that long-lasting pain relief with preservation of structural integrity of bone would be of major concern. As a general rule, when shorter courses of radiotherapy are shown to yield the same response rate, they are to be preferred. Other factors that can influence the choice of fractionation include the duration of response, acute side effects, chronic complications and the retreatment rate.

BONE METASTASES

PATHOLOGY & CLINICAL FEATURES

Autopsy studies of cancer patients have demonstrated bone metastases in up to 70% of patients. Cancers of the breast, prostate, lung, thyroid and kidney metastasize to bone quite frequently. Less commonly, primary tumors of the pancreas, cervix, stomach, colon, ovary and esophagus as well as melanomas and lymphomas will spread to bone.

Presenting symptoms may include bone pain, spontaneous pathologic fracture, and neurologic symptoms related to compression of the spinal cord, cranial nerves or peripheral nerves from extraosseous extension of tumor or bony collapse.

WORK-UP

When bone metastases are suspected on the basis of history and physical examination, the radionuclide bone scan is the most sensitive test. It will show increased uptake in metastatic deposits long before there is the requisite 50% bony destruction to yield a discrete osteolytic lesion on plain radiographs. A skeletal survey, including orthogonal views of both femurs, is necessary to detect other bony lesions with potential for pathologic fracture in weight bearing bones. Radiographically, bone metastases may be osteolytic, osteoblastic or mixed. Their radiographic appearance may be related to the tumor growth kinetics. Slower growing tumors such as prostate induce condensation of bone, while rapidly growing tumors such as lung produce lytic changes. In multiple myeloma there may be significant radiographic bone destruction in areas that are not positive on a bone scan, since some new bone formation must be present to demonstrate increased uptake on bone scan.

Bone biopsy is occasionally necessary to (1) establish a tissue diagnosis in the case of bone metastases of unknown primary site and (2) to document metastatic disease in patients whose primary malignancy has been controlled prior to the initiation of potentially toxic therapy. Useful laboratory studies include: serum calcium, alkaline phosphatase and acid phosphatase (prostate).

TREATMENT AND RESULTS

Surgery

Bone metastases causing greater than 50% destruction of the cortex place the patient at increased risk for pathologic fracture. When long bones are involved, orthopedic consultation should be sought and prophylactic fixation using an intramedullary rod or plates should be considered, again depending on the patient's performance status and surgical risk. In patients who are unsuitable for general anesthesia, impending fractures of the femur can prophylactically be stablized using Ender nails with a local anesthetic. Results comparable to those achieved with open fixation have been claimed. The advantages of initial surgical management include pain relief, prevention of pathologic fracture, and early mobilization which is important to prevent hypercalcemia and decubitus ulcers. When operative fixation is carried out, postoperative radiotherapy is recommended to control the underlying cancer.

Medical Therapy

Hormonal manipulation will provide pain relief in many patients with metastatic prostate or breast cancers. Occasionally, bone pain will respond to systemic chemotherapy.

Radiation Therapy

Involved field radiotherapy: A long held tenet of radiotherapy has been to treat the entire bone when it is involved with metastatic disease. However, such patients are often receiving combination chemotherapy and this principle must be tempered by the need to conserve bone marrow. A variety of dose fractionation schemes ranging from large single fractions (500-1200 rad) to 5000 rad over five weeks have been shown effective in the palliation of bone metastases in several retrospective studies. The RTOG has investigated the utility of several of these treatment schemes in randomized prospective studies. A dose of 3000 rad in 10 fractions over two weeks was found to be optimum. Shorter fractionation schemes have resulted in a somewhat higher retreatment rate. Permanent significant pain relief can be expected in up to 80% of patients treated. Several authors have observed that prostate cancer responds somewhat more slowly.

Hemi-body irradiation: Patients with multiple sites of metastases, whose dominant sites of painful bony metastases include the ribs, shoulder girdle, cervicothoracic spine and skull may be treated with large anterior and posterior fields encompassing the upper hemi-body using the superior aspect of the iliac crest as the lower margin of the field. Because of the inclusion of the upper abdomen and lungs within the treatment fields, it is necessary to premedicate patients with a regimen of hydration, corticosteroids and antinauseants to prevent nausea and hypotension. The parotid gland should be blocked from the treatment portal to prevent xerostomia. If there is no skull involvement, the head may be excluded to avoid alopecia. Single midplane doses ranging from 600 to 800 rad are given. It is necessary to compensate for the increased dose to the lungs which is due to increased transmission through the less dense pulmonary parenchyma. The dose to the lungs is also affected by the energy of the treatment machine with a higher dose given from a 10 MeV linear accelerator compared with cobalt teletherapy. If corrections for lung density and treatment machine characteristics cannot be made, the given dose should be limited to 700 rad.

Lower hemi-body irradiation can be utilized when there are extensive symptomatic bony metastases involving the lumbar spine, pelvis and lower extremities. Premedication is usually unneccessary since the hypotension associated with upper hemi-body irradiation has not been observed. Single doses of 800 to 1000 rad may be given.

The use of hemi-body irradiation often produces dramatic pain relief within 48 hours following treatment in up to 70% of patients. Results tend to be more favorable and of longer duration in patients with indolent "chronic" cancers. Because of the rapidity of pain relief, it is possible that the immediate response may be mediated through release of endogenous opiates (endorphins and enkephalins) since objective tumor regression could not have yet occurred.

MORBIDITY

Bone marrow: Irradiation of more than 50% of the bone marrow can result in a clinically significant depression of peripheral blood counts. Lymphocytes are the most sensitive of the formed elements. They are one of very few cell types which undergo an interphase death. Other mature blood elements are radioresistant and decline according to their half-lifes due to stem cell damage by radiation. When segments of bone marrow are irradiated, long-term severe marrow depopulation occurs at doses of 4000 rad and above. At 2000 rad to a segment of bone marrow significant recovery occurs at 1 year.

Other: The toxicity of radiotherapy for bone metastases is generally related to other tissues included in the radiation portal. If there is a significant amount of bowel within the treatment volume, nausea and diarrhea can be seen. For upper hemi-body irradiation, an acute radiation syndrome consisting of nausea, chills, vomiting, fever, tachycardia and hypotension is possible but can be prevented by the use of a premedication program as described above. For lower hemi-body irradiation nausea occurs in about a third of patients and vomiting in one-sixth. In patients who have received prior radiotherapy, however, postirradiation osteitis may masquerade as metastatic disease.

MENINGEAL TUMOR INFILTRATION

PATHOLOGY & CLINICAL FEATURES

Infiltration of the meninges with tumor leads to obstruction of cerebrospinal fluid (CSF) flow or subsequent invasion of brain, spinal cord or nerve. This can lead to increased intracranial pressure, hydrocephalus, seizure, hemiparesis or multifocal neurologic deficits.

Meningeal infiltrate occurs most commonly in ALL but also is seen in lymphomas and carcinomas, particularly adenocarcinoma of the breast or lung. As effective chemotherapy yields prolonged survival, especially in lymphomatous and hematologic malignancy, meningeal tumor infiltration is being recognized with increased frequency.

WORK-UP

The diagnosis is suggested by widespsread findings including cranial nerve deficits on neurologic examination. CSF should be examined for cytology, increased pressure, increased protein or decreased glucose. The initial tap yields positive cytology in less than 50% of patients; thus, several taps may be needed. A myelogram should be performed to rule out gross tumor deposits that may cause extradural compression.

TREATMENT AND RESULTS

Treatment must be directed to the entire neuraxis. Radiation is directed only to areas of gross deposits or extradural compression seen on myelogram. Treatment should be given immediately after diagnosis is established. Most medical oncologists advocate intrathecal administration of methotrexate over systemic therapy. Drugs can be given via lumbar puncture or intraventricularly via the Ommaya device. If drugs are administered by lumbar puncture, consideration of whole brain irradiation should be given since drug distribution over the cerebral convexities is often inadequate. Radiation doses and fractionation are variable with histology; however, generally they are in the 2000-4000 rad in 2-4 weeks.

Untreated patients usually succumb within 6 months of diagnosis. Patients with leukemia or lymphoma usually respond quite well with improvement in neurologic symptoms. Often CNS disease is controlled until they succumb from systemic disease. Breast and lung cancers respond moderately well with more than 50% of patients having neurologic improvement.

MORBIDITY

Treatment complications are related primarily to drug toxicity (asceptic meningitis, necrotizing leukoencephalopathy) or to Ommaya reservoir placement (infection). Necrotizing leukoencephalopathy occurs most frequently when radiation is given in conjunction with intraventricular or systemic methotrexate. In order to avoid this, whole brain radiation should not be given if methotrexate is administered through an Ommaya reservoir or systemically at high doses.

BRAIN METASTASES

PATHOLOGY & CLINICAL FEATURES

Neurologic deficits from brain metastases result from either obstruction to CSF flow or from compression and disturbances in the environment of surrounding normal brain tissue.

Over 25% of all patients presenting with brain tumors have, in fact, brain metastases. Lung, breast, kidney, melanoma and G.I. malignancies represent the most common primary tumor sites which metastasize to the brain. The majority of brain metastases are multiple, with only 20% being solitary.

The rapidity of progression of neurologic dysfunction is quite variable and depends upon location and aggressiveness of the metastases. More than 50% of patients with brain metastases present with headache. Characteristically the headache is mild, presenting in the early morning and diminishing approximately one-half hour after arising. Papilledema is found on presentation in only 25% of patients.

WORK-UP

The most sensitive and accurate test for diagnosing brain metastases is the CT scan. Although the distinctions are not always clear-cut, the CT scan is useful in differentiating intracranial hemorrhage, thrombosis, cystic masses and abscess from solid tumor with edema. Lumbar puncture is not performed unless meningeal tumor is suspected and increased intracranial pressure has been treated.

TREATMENT

Approximately 75% of patients will experience some short-lived degree of symptomatic relief from dexamethasone administration alone. All patients should be started on dexamethasone prior to initiation of radiation therapy. The dose usually is $\geq$16 mg/day and can be tapered to the lowest dose which relieves symptoms. If the patient is noted to have rapid clinical deterioration and cerebral herniation is impending, a rapid decrease in intracranial pressure can be effected through the use of mannitol (I.V.) or glycerol (p.o.). If the patient had seizures as a presenting symptom, phenytoin 300-400 mg/day is recommended. The prophylactic use of phenytoin (in patients without prior history of seizures) is not widely accepted due to: (1) the difficulty in differentiating tumor recurrence from drug toxicity, (2) changes in drug metabolism due to phenytoin's stimulation of the hepatic microsomal system, and (3) increased risk (though rare) of Stevens-Johnson syndrome when brain radiation and phenytoin are given together.

Surgery may be indicated in patients presenting with a solitary site of brain metastasis if there has been a greater than one year disease-free interval. Furthermore, the tumor should be accessible so that postoperative morbidity is minimized. Other possible indications for surgical therapy include: (1) uncertain diagnosis, (2) failure of nonsurgical therapy, and (3) relatively radioresistant solitary metastases from melanomas or sarcomas. Radiation therapy should follow surgical excision.

Radiation therapy remains the treatment of choice for the majority of patients. The whole brain is treated to doses of 2000-4000 rad in 1-3 weeks.

RESULTS

Without treatment the median survival is approximately one month. Use of steroids alone increases the median survival to approximately 2 months. In patients with single metastasis undergoing surgical extirpation followed by radiation therapy, median survival is approximately 5-6 months with approximately 25% surviving one year. The median survival for patients treated with radiation therapy alone is approximately 4-6 months. Approximately 60% of patients treated with radiation therapy alone experience neurologic improvement lasting 3-6 months. The quality of survival is no better following surgical extirpation than that following radiation therapy.

MORBIDITY

Acute

Whole brain irradiation is associated with temporary alopecia after 2000-3000 rad. Skin erythema and tiredness may also occur.

Chronic

Permanent alopecia may be induced with high doses of radiation, particularly if systemic chemotherapy is also given. (See Chapter 5 for other CNS morbidity) Brain necrosis from radiation is not seen after doses typically given for brain metastases (e.g. 3000 rad/2 weeks). There is no evidence that radiation at this dose impairs intellectual function in adults.

HEPATIC METASTASES

PATHOLOGY & CLINICAL FEATURES

With its extensive network of sinusoids, the liver presents the first vascular sieve to filter venous blood from the remainder of the intra-abdominal gastro-intestinal tract. Therefore, the most common hepatic metastases are from cancers of these organs: colon, rectum, stomach, esophagus and pancreas. Other tumors that frequently metastasize to liver include breast, lung, melanoma, lymphoma, ovary, bladder and other genitourinary tumors.

Liver metastases are a common finding in patients with end-stage cancer, being present in 50-75% of these patients at autopsy. The symptoms of hepatic metastases include pain, nausea, vomiting, anorexia, jaundice and ascites. Occasionally, hepatic metastasis will be the initial manifestation of a malignancy or the cause of fever of unknown origin.

WORK-UP

When hepatic metastases are suspected, liver function tests including alkaline phosphatase, gamma glutamyl transpeptidase, SGOT, SGPT, bilirubin, albumin and prothrombin time are useful. A physical examination often discloses hepatomegaly with a nodular liver edge. Friction rubs may be audible over the liver. A technetium 99m sulfur colloid liver scan is capable of resolving focal defects greater than 2 cm in diamter. Abdominal CT scans and ultrasonography are useful, complementary, non-invasive tests for the detection of hepatic metastases. Blind percutaneous needle biopsy has a false-negative rate of up to 50%. This yield can be improved somewhat when the biopsy procedure is guided by peritoneoscopy or CT. When present, jaundice may be due to either diffuse parenchymal metastatic disease or extra-hepatic biliary tract obstruction from metastatic tumor near the porta hepatis. Transhepatic cholangiography in the jaundiced patient is useful in the differential diagnosis, and may provide accurate localization of the obstruction for the radiation therapist.

TREATMENT AND RESULTS

Surgery

Partial hepatectomy may be considered in selected patients with solitary metastases, yielding a five-year survival up to 30%. Patients with multiple hepatic metastases fare less well. The 17% operative mortality rate exceeds the five-year survival rate of 14%. Hepatic artery ligation can result in palliation of symptoms in 50-60% of patients, although survival does not appear to be prolonged.

Systemic Chemotherapy

The use of 5-FU in the treatment of liver metastases from colorectal cancer results in a 20-30% response rate. The median duration of response is 3-5 months with no significant survival benefit. Intrahepatic arterial chemotherapeutic infusions have been used since 1950. The rationales for this approach are:

1. Metastases derive their blood supply from the hepatic artery.
2. Higher tumor concentrations can be achieved.
3. Systemic side effects are minimized by hepatic metabolism and clearance of the infused drugs.

Response rates vary from 30-80% with median survivals in responders to intra-arterial chemotherapy being as high as 16 months. A prospective randomized study comparing intra-arterial chemotherapy with systemic chemotherapy failed to substantiate a survival advantage. Complications related to catheter insertion or dislodgement during infusion occur in 10-40% of patients. With the recent development of implantable infusion pumps capable of exposing tumors to continuous low levels of chemotherapeutic agents without prolonged hospitalization, intra-arterial administration will need to re-examined.

Radiotherapy

Hepatic irradiation will produce significant pain relief, reduction in hepatomegaly and improvement in liver function tests in 55-95% of patients treated. Fractionation schemes range from 2100-2400 rad in 7-8 fractions over a two week period to 2800 rad in 14 treatments. The median survivals in several series range from 4-6 months, only slightly better than the median survival of 75 days in cases of untreated liver metastases of diverse histology. Patients with an objective response to treatment have a 9 month median survival.

Several efforts have been made to improve the palliative effect and objective response rate from radiation therapy. These include the addition of hypoxic cell sensitizers such as Misonidazole, which as yet has proved unrewarding. Another effort is the combined use of intra-arterial chemotherapy plus total hepatic irradiation. Pilot studies are encouraging with median survivals for the entire treated group of about 8 months. A prospective randomized study to determine the place of such a combined-modality approach is warranted.

MORBIDITY

Acute

Surprisingly, hepatic irradiation is quite well tolerated with mild nausea seen in 20% and severe nausea in only 10%.

Chronic

The liver is a radiosensitive organ but radiation hepatitis is rare below doses of 3000 rad. (See Chapter 10)

The risk of radiation nephritis exists when treating the liver since the right kidney is generally included in the treatment portals. This can be avoided by shielding the kidney after a dose of 1500-1800 rad. Alternatively, it may be possible to exclude the right kidney from the treatment by using oblique fields.

METASTATIC NON-SQUAMOUS CANCER OF UNKNOWN ORIGIN

OVERVIEW

Not infrequently, the first manifestation of malignant disease is the appearance of distant metastases, with this presentation constituting 3-10% of all cancer patients. Sites of involvement may include regional lymph nodes, viscera, skeleton or integument. The management of metastatic squamous cell carcinoma involving cervical lymph nodes of unknown primary site is discussed in Chapter 4.

PATHOLOGY

When viscera, bone or integument are involved, the primary sites are most often lung, pancreas, stomach, colon, liver and kidney, none of which are particularly treatable in their metastatic presentation. Metastatic adenocarcinomas or undifferentiated carcinomas may originate from the breast in axillary presentations or from the GI tract and lung, in supraclavicular presentations. The role of the pathologist is to aid in the search for a primary tumor which may be responsive to hormonal management or chemotherapy such as breast cancer, prostate cancer, variants of small cell lung cancer, lymphoma and germ cell tumors. In this regard, special stains, immunohistochemical evaluation, electron microscopy and assays for hormone receptors may be appropriate. Determination of beta HCG subunits and alpha fetoprotein should be carried out in patients presenting with undifferentiated malignancies of the lung and mediastinum since these patients may represent "the unrecognized extra-gonadal germ cell cancer syndrome". If a diagnosis of malignant lymphoma is considered, immune surface markers for B and T cell differentiation can be carried out.

WORK-UP

A thorough history and physical exam including pelvic, breast and rectal exams are indispensible. A chest x-ray, CBC, urinalysis, chemical profiles and proctosigmoidoscopy are generally agreed to be routine. Several reported series have employed extensive contrast radiographic searches including upper GI series, barium enema, IVP and mammography as well as extensive radionuclide scanning. Some authors now feel that these procedures are not only of low yield but may also be misleading and should not be used routinely. The work-up should be individualized and other techniques such as abdominal ultrasound, CT scanning and gallium scanning be used judiciously. Time consumption, patient comfort and cost should be considered when designing an individual work-up. Despite extensive work-ups, the primary cancer site can be established in only 10-20% of patients.

TREATMENT AND RESULTS

For patients presenting with extensive metastatic cancer of unknown origin, the median survival ranges from 2-7 months. If the patient is asymptomatic, observation alone is reasonable. If a more treatable disease such as lymphoma, extra-gonadal germ cell tumor, breast cancer or ovarian cancer cannot be ruled out, a chemotherapeutic regimen known to be effective in these tumors should be considered. Likewise, additive hormonal therapy is reasonable when prostatic, breast and ovarian carcinoma cannot be excluded. The empiric use of 5-FU based chemotherapeutic regimens has been unrewarding with response rates of 4-12%. In this population, radiotherapy should be reserved for palliation of specific symptoms. Women who present with adenocarcinoma involving an axillary node with an unknown primary should be managed as though they had occult breast cancer. Since the breast disease can be assumed to be subclinical (no palpable mass and negative mammography) irradiation of the breast and peripheral lymphatics to 5000 rad in 5 weeks will yield local control in most patients. Montague reports a 50% NED survival in 8 patients so treated.

REFERENCES

1. Richter MP: Palliative radiation therapy. In Cassileth BR and Cassileth PA (eds): Clinical Care of the Terminal Patient, Philadelphia, Lea & Febiger, 1982, p 65.
2. Tong D, Gillick L and Hendrickson FR: The palliation of symptomatic osseous metastases. Cancer 50:893-899, 1982.
3. Salazar OM et al: Single-dose half-body irradiation for the palliation of multiple bone metastases from solid tumors: a preliminary report. I J Rad Onc Bio Phys 7:773-781, 1981.
4. Borgelt B et al: The palliation of brain metastases: final results of the first two studies by the radiation therapy oncology group. I J Rad Onc Bio Phys 6:1-9, 1979.
5. Posner J: Management of central nervous system metastases. Semin Oncol 14:1977.
6. Hendrickson FR et al: The influence of surgery and radiation therapy on patients with brain metastases. I J Rad Onc Bio Phys 9:623-627, 1982.
7. Borgelt B et al: The palliation of hepatic metastases: results of the Radiation Therapy Oncology Group pilot study. I J Rad Onc Bio Phys 7:587-592, 1981.
8. Neumann KH, Nystrom JS: Metastatic cancer of unknown origin: nonsquamous cell type. Semin Oncol 9:427-434, 1982.

Chapter 18

Combined-Modality

OVERVIEW

With notable exceptions, a therapeutic radiologist can rarely expect to achieve local control when bulky tumors are treated with radiotherapy following only an incisional biopsy. These exceptions include Hodgkin's and non-Hodgkin's lymphoma, plasmacytoma, Ewing's sarcoma and seminoma. Table 18.1 shows the doses required to control macroscopic deposits of squamous and adenocarcinomas. This sobering fact is the rationale behind combined-modality management of cancer. Both surgery and radiotherapy are local treatments; however, cancer is often not a local disease. Thus, the stage is set for systemic therapy to further improve local control and survival. In this chapter strategies for combined modality treatment will be discussed. Ways in which surgeons, radiotherapists and medical oncologists can maximize gain to the patient by effectively working together and anticipating the special needs of each discipline will be outlined. Specific examples of collaborative efforts can be found in most chapters throughout the book, but head and neck may serve as a model. Potential toxicities of combined approaches will also be discussed.

SURGERY AND RADIOTHERAPY

Surgery can be combined with radiotherapy in four fashions:

Preoperative radiotherapy has as its goals (a) to increase the resectability rate for bulky tumors by reducing their size, (b) to diminish the viability of tumor cells that can be implanted in the surgical bed at the time of the operation and (c) to diminish the number of viable cells that have access to the circulatory system and thus reduce the chances for distant metastases. The advantage of this approach is that the irradiated tissues are better vascularized and oxygenated prior to surgery. The preoperative radiation

Table 18.1 (from Fletcher & Schukovsky)
Probability of Control Correlated with Irradiation Dose and Volume of Cancer

Dose	Squamous Cell Carcinoma of the Upper Respiratory and Digestive Tracts	Adenocarcinoma of the Breast
5000 rad[a]	>90% subclinical 50% T1 lesions of nasopharynx ≅50% 2-3 cm neck nodes	>90% subclinical
6000 rad[a]	80-90% T1 lesions of pharynx and larynx ≅50% T3 + T4 lesions of tonsillar fossa	
7000 rad[a]	≅90% 1-3 cm neck nodes ≅70% 3-5 cm neck nodes 80-90% T2 lesions of tonsillar fossa and supraglottic larynx ≅80% T3 + T4 lesions of tonsillar fossa	90% clinically positive axillary nodes 2.5-3 cm[b]
7000-8000 rad (8-9 weeks)		65% 2-3 cm primary 30% >5 cm primary
8000-9000 rad (8-10 weeks)		56% >5 cm primary
8000-10,000 rad (10-12 weeks)		75% >5-15 cm primary

[a] 1000 rad/5 fractions/1 week.

[b] The control rate is corrected for the percentage of nodes that would be positive histologically had a dissection of the axilla been performed.

[c] Data from Fletcher and Schukovsky, 1975.[10]

dose and the time interval between radiotherapy and surgery depends upon the weight that is placed upon each of the above stated goals. If the main concern is to prevent implantation and reduce metastatic potential, a lower dose or shorter course with immediate surgery may be elected. However, if the main goal is to make a marginally resectable or unresectable lesion amenable to surgery by "downstaging", a higher dose and a longer waiting period (3-6 weeks) would be more rational. The disadvantages of preoperative irradiation are interference with wound healing, and delay in curative surgery. Preoperative radiotherapy has been used with success in the management of head and neck tumors, soft tissue sarcomas, superior sulcus lung tumors and rectal cancer. Because of the inaccuracy of clinical staging, some low-risk patients may receive preoperative radiotherapy if it is applied routinely.

Postoperative radiotherapy is indicated when complete resection of cancer either at the primary site or the regional lymphatics has been incomplete or improbable. In general, specific indications include extensive lymph node metastases especially with extracapsular extension, inadequate or postive surgerical margins, and certain high-grade, deeply-invasive tumors which place the regional lymphatics at significant risk for occult metastatic disease. The advantages of postoperative irradiation are that precise pathologic staging is available, the extent of the tumor is known, allowing accurate design of the radiaiton portals, and wound healing can be completed. Disadvantages are that contamination of the surgical bed by tumor spillage can force the radiotherapist to design rather large portals to encompass sites of potential disease and the formation of scar tissue creates a hypoxic milieu making residual cancer more radioresistant. Traditionally, postoperative irradiation has been used extensively in the treatment of brain tumors, head and neck cancer, breast cancer, lung cancer, gastrointestinal lymphomas, rectal cancer, gynecologic malignancies (ovary and endometrium) and soft tissue sarcomas.

"Selective sandwich" radiotherapy seems an ideal solution to many of the problems of both pre and postoperative radiotherapy. This technique involves the delivery of a single high fractional preoperative dose (500-800 rad) to the tumor bed with the goal of reducing the clonogenic potential of 80-90% of the well-oxygenated tumor cells, which may be shed at the time of surgery. This does not delay extirpation of tumor which is often comforting to both patient and surgeon. On the basis of careful pathologic staging, full dose postoperative radiotherapy can be given to the surgical bed and regional lymphatics in high-risk patients. Pilot studies of this technique in the management of rectal cancer have been conducted at Thomas Jefferson University Hospital and Massachusetts General Hospital, suggesting the efficacy of this approach. "Sandwich" radiotherapy is now the subject of a randomized phase III RTOG study for rectal cancer. Other sites where the "sandwich" has been applied include bladder cancer and intrathoracic malignancies.

Salvage surgery following full therapeutic doses of radiation is another option that the oncology team will occasionally consider. This is rational in the case of head and neck tumors where radical surgery will result in a substantial cosmetic or functional defect. An example is locally advanced laryngeal carcinoma. If radiotherapy is successful, the patient will have preservation of speech. If radiotherapy fails, radical surgery can then be performed for salvage. One would expect a higher surgical morbidity since the tissue has received doses in the order of 6600-7000 rad. However, an RTOG study (73-03) found that there was no statistically significant increase in morbidity, with comparable survival rates.

INTERACTION BETWEEN SURGEON & RADIOTHERAPIST

Whenever there is even a remote possibility of a combined-modality surgical-radiotherapeutic approach to a particular cancer patient, presurgical evaluation by the radiotherapist is beneficial because it allows the radiotherapist to appreciate the extent of tumor. In the case of gastrointestinal malignancies, the radiotherapist can advise the surgeon of his anticipated treatment portals so that it may be possible to place internal anastomoses outside the high dose volume and cutaneous ostomies out of the fields. A detailed operative note is invaluable. It should include a description of the size of the tumor and its anatomic extent, noting of fixation or invasion of adjacent structures, whether or not regional lymph nodes are palpable and suspicious for malignancy. It is likewise important if distant metastases were suspected on the basis of palpation or inspection (e.g. liver). Histologic confirmation is essential since the patient is usually deemed incurable and any further aggressive local postoperative radiotherapy would be inappropriate. If a tumor is unresectable (e.g. pancreas), the mass should be outlined with clips including the posterior margin. These will serve as a guide for postoperative radiotherapy and will allow the radiotherapist to minimize the volume of normal tissue that will be irradiated. Also, if a margin of resection is felt to be inadequate, this should also be marked with clips for a possible boost using shrinking field techniques. Finally, it is often helpful for radiotherapists to review postoperative radiographs and simulator films with the surgeon prior to the initiation of treatment as a means of defining the tumor volume.

In patients who have received prior radiotherapy and will need surgery either as part of the neoplastic management or for complications or unrelated illnesses, presurgical consultation with the radiotherapist is essential. Treatment portals often permanently marked with skin tatoos can be outlined. The type and dose of radiotherapy with its expected effects on the skin and subcutaneous tissue can be defined. This information may aid the surgeon in his choice of a particular bowel segment for an anastomosis or influence his decision regarding the use of stay sutures. In the case of soft tissue sarcomas of the extremities, the placement of a biopsy incision is of critical importance since it should be encompassed in a pre or postoperative radiation portal. To minimize post-irradiation morbidity, it is important that the entire circumference of the limb not be irradiated. A poorly placed incision can make this technically very difficult.

MORBIDITY OF COMBINED SURGERY & RADIOTHERAPY

The main problems using a combined approach of surgery and radiotherapy relate to wound healing because of interference with cellular proliferation. Delayed wound healing, soft tissue necrosis and wound breakdown can be seen with increased frequency. These complications can be minimized by meticulous surgical techniques. Irradiated tissues should be handled delicately with particular attention to hemostasis. Depending on the dose, the combination of abdominal irradiation and surgery can lead to increased incidences of adhesions, anastomotic leaks, fistulous tracts and intestinal obstruction. When the lymph node dissections of the axillary or inguinal content are combined with radiotherapy, distal edema and fibrosis are not uncommon. When a combined approach is anticipated in managing regional lymph nodes, classical radical lymphadenectomies in the head and neck and axilla can be modified to less extensive, less morbid procedures.

CHEMOTHERAPY AND RADIOTOHERAPY

In the last two decades, the number of chemotherapeutic agents and their efficacy against advanced malignancies has increased dramatically. Systemic chemotherapy may now be combined with radiotherapy in almost unlimited number of permutations. Three such ways predominate and will serve to illustrate the principles involved:

Chemotherapy given prior to radiotherapy and/or surgery has proven valuable in "debulking" massive primary tumors in the head and neck region, the breast and for bone and soft tissue sarcomas, often converting unresectable lesions into one that can be managed successfully by surgery or radiotherapy. This use has been termed induction or neoadjuvant chemotherapy. The rationale for this approach is that (1) the intact vascularity allows for optimal drug delivery, (2) performance status and nutrition are generally better prior to any radiotherapy or surgery and this allows for improved tolerance of aggressive chemotherapy and (3) there is no delay in the treatment of occult metastases. The experience with locally advanced head and neck tumors is illustrative. Major response rates for induction chemotherapy have ranged from 52-97%. In the head and neck experience there has been no obvious increase in morbidity from either subsequent surgery or radiation.

<u>Chemotherapy given concomitantly with radiotherapy</u> is employed in two situations: (1) the treatment of bulky tumors with the goal of obtaining a synergistic or supra-additive effect capitalizing on the <u>radio-sensitizing</u> properties of some chemotherapeutic agents. Agents which appear to be radiosensitizers include doxorubicin, 5-FU, bleomycin, hydroxyurea, methotrexate, cisplatin and actinomycin-D. Examples where concomitant therapy has been employed are unresectable head and neck tumors and unresectable bronchogenic carcinoma (including small cell). Another situation in which concomitant management is indicated is for tumors where adjuvant therapy has been successful in preventing or delaying distant metastases and where delay in initiation of such therapy while the primary tumor is being managed radiotherapeutically is felt to be detrimental. Specifically, this is the case in stage II breast cancer where either radiotherapy is being employed as primary management following lumpectomy or as an adjuvant following mastectomy in cetain patients with high risk for chest wall recurrence. Several investigators have reported the ability to give full dose chemotherapy during breast or chest wall irradiation with acceptable skin and soft tissue morbidity and little hematologic toxicity.

<u>Chemotherapy after primary surgical or radiotherapeutic management of the primary tumor</u> is given adjuvantly to sterilize micrometastases which may be present at the time of diagnosis. The success of this approach has been demonstrated for stage II breast cancer, soft tissue sarcomas and several pediatric solid tumors.

A "sandwich" technique interdigitating radiotherapy between cycles of chemotherapy is sometimes employed in diseases such as Hodgkin's disease and small cell lung cancer which are very sensitive to chemotherapy, yet have a predilection to recur at the original sites of bulk disease. With this technique, induction chemotherapy will produce complete or partial tumor regression after two or three drug cycles. Moderate dose radiotherapy is then employed to consolidate the remission. This is followed by a maintenance phase of chemotherapy.

MORBIDITY OF COMBINATIONS OF CHEMOTHERAPY & RADIOTHERAPY

Acute

Exacerbation of skin reaction has been reported with the concomitant use of actinomycin-D, 5-FU, bleomycin, hydroxurea and methotrexate. Mucositis may be enhanced by concomitant use of 5-FU and methotrexate. No such enhancement has been reported with the combined use of cisplatin and radiation. Prior mediastinal irradiation appears to be a risk factor for adriamycin induced cardiomyopathy. Mediastinal irradiation for esophageal or lung cancer causes esophagitis which will be increased when drugs such as bleomycin, actinomycin-D, methotrexate, vinca alkaloids and doxorubicin are given during or shortly after radiotherapy. A "recall esophagitis" has been described in patients receiving adriamycin following radiotherapy. Bleomycin appears to be a potent sensitizer of pulmonary parenchymal damage from therapeutic doses of radiation given for bronchogenic carcinoma. Severe radiation pneumonitis has also been reported with doxorubicin, actinomycin-D, vincristine, procarbazine and hydroxurea. Gastrointestinal toxicity is exacerbated by the concomitant use of 5-FU, mitomycin-C, doxorubicin and actinomycin-D. Radiation nephritis will occur at a lower radiation dose when concomitant actinomycin-D is employed. Combined cranial irradiation and methotrexate (either given systemically or intrathecally) has been shown to cause leukoencephalopathy in the setting of ALL.

Chronic

A feared complication of multidisciplinary management of various malignancies is the appearance of second primary tumors, very often hematologic malignancies. This is seen with increasing frequency in several diseases where treatment has produced long-term disease-free survival. In Hodgkin's disease, patient's treated with combined radiation-chemotherapy, the risk of developing late second neoplasms is approximately 7-10%. The use of alkylating agents has been implicated in this problem. Other sites where this problem has been reported include small cell lung cancer, ovarian cancer and high grade gliomas.

REFERENCES

1. Durant JR: Future of combined modality therapy. I J Rad Onc Bio Phys 7:783-790, 1981.
2. Glick JH, Taylor SG: Integration of chemotherapy into a combined modality treatment plan for head and neck cancer: a review. I J Rad Onc Bio Phys 7:229-242, 1981.
3. Mohiuddin M, Kramer S et al: Combined pre and postoperative radiation for carcinoma of the rectum. I J Rad Onc Bio Phys 8:133-136, 1981.
4. Cummings BJ et al: Combined radical radiation therapy and chemotherapy for primary squamous cell carcinoma of the anal canal. Cancer Treatment Reports 66:489-492, 1982.

Chapter 19

Radiation Safety

OVERVIEW

Because of the biologic delay between radiation exposure and the expression of damage, there are no early warning signs of moderate exposure. Since ionizing radiation cannot be perceived by the five senses, certain precautions must be taken to alert humans of potential exposure. In this chapter the basic principles of radiation protection will be outlined as they apply to house officers charged with the care of patients who are receiving intravenous radioisotopes, or intracavitary or interstitial radioactive implants as part of their antineoplastic management.

RISK OF LOW DOSE RADIATION

The existence of a threshold for the biologic effects of low dose radiation is disputed. Extrapolation of data obtained at much higher doses may very likely lead to an overestimation of the risk of low levels of radiation to man. The conservative approach of estimating radiation exposure risk assumes:

1. That possible effects at extremely low doses are directly related to known consequences at higher doses (linear hypothesis).
2. That any amount of of radiation involves some risk (no threshold exists).
3. That several small doses at intervals has a cumulative effect equal to the sum delivered as a single dose.
4. That there is no repair of radiation injury.

It is doubtful that this controversy will ever be resolved experimentally since radiation effects at low doses are so small that vast number of animals would need to be tested to prove injury produced by exposure of only a few roentgens. Because of this uncertainty every effort should be taken to minimize exposure of patients and health personnel to sources of ionizing radiation.

DOSE EQUIVALENT

The rem (roentgen equivalent man) is a traditional unit used by therapeutic radiologists and medical physicists in measurements referring to radiation protection and allows for comparison of effects of different types of radiation.

REM = amount of energy absorbed (RAD) x the efficiency of radiation in producing damage (quality factor = QF)

$$REM = RAD \times QF$$

The quality factor (qf) accounts for the different degree of damage produced by equal doses of different types of radiation. The quality factor for photons and beta particles is one; therefore, the rem and the rad in this case are equivalent and are used interchangably. For neutrons, the quality factor will range from 2 to 10 depending upon neutron energy; while the quality factor for alpha particles may range from 10 to 20. The SI (international) unit for dose equivalent is the sievert.

1 rem = 1000 mrem
100 rem = 1 sievert (Sv)

LATE EFFECTS OF IONIZING RADIATION

The three principle late effects of concern are (1) non-specific life shortening, (2) carcinogenesis and (3) genetic and teratogenic effects.

Non-specific life shortening has not been clearly demonstrated in humans, although there is definite evidence for this effect in animal studies.

Carcinogenesis and leukemogenesis have long been recognized as hazards of radiation exposure. Skin cancer was an occupational hazard for early radiologists and physicists. Survivors of Hiroshima and Nagasaki have also had an increased incidence of leukemia and other cancers. The development of post-radiation neoplasms is characterized by a latent period, which may be as little as 5 years for leukemias and up to 25 years for solid tumors. Epidemiologic studies have shown an excess of leukemia and other cancers in children who have been irradiated in utero when their mothers were exposed to diagnostic x-ray procedures. It is estimated that prenatal irradiation may increase the risk of malignancy during the first 10 years of life by twofold.

Genetic and teratogenic effects must be inferred from animal experimentation, since there is little direct evidence to estimate the genetic hazards of radiation exposure in man. Again, a conservative approach is warranted and assumes that no matter how small a dose of radiation some genetic risk is involved. An attempt to estimate the exposure that is relevant to mutation production, the genetically significant dose (GSD), has been described as an index of the presumed genetic impact to radiation on the whole population. The GSD for the whole population is the dose expected to result in the same total genetic injury to the population as the actual gonadal doses received by various individuals exposed. In a 1970 survey by the U.S. Bureau of Radiologic Health, the GSD for diagnostic radiology procedures was 20 mrad, which compared with 90 mrad due to natural background levels. Occupational exposure accounted for only 0.8 mrad.

The effect of ionizing radiation on the embryo or fetus depends on the dose and development period. The in utero developmental period can be divided into preimplantation stage, organogenesis and fetal stage. Exposure during preimplantation results in a high incidence of prenatal death; however, if the embryo survives it is likely to develop normally without any growth retardation. During organogenesis radiation exposure leads to congenital malformations (teratogenesis) and intrauterine growth retardation. During the fetal stage, congenital malformations are less likely to occur. Some permanent growth retardation and possible mental retardation is possible from radiation exposure during this period.

EXPOSURE TO IONIZING RADIIATION

Man is constantly exposed to evironmental sources of radiation, both natural and manmade.

Table 19.1
Natural Background Exposure

Source	Average Dose
Sun, cosmic rays	30-40 mrem/year
Radioactive material in the earth's crust	40 mrem/year
Radon in the air, radioactive potassium in food & water	25-30 mrem/year

The geographic location of one's residence can dramatically affect yearly exposure. For instance, a person dwelling in the coastal plains would have approximately 60-70 mrem exposure/year, while a person living on a mountain plateau would receive up to 165 mrem/year because of the increased altitude with increased exposure to cosmic rays. However, no increase in cancers has been attributed to this difference in exposure.

Manmade Exposure

The largest manmade contribution of the average radiation exposure in the United States is from the medical use of ionizing radiation. Medical exposure is usually a partial body exposure given over a short period, thus making comparison with background exposure partially misleading. Nevertheless, one can compare the average bone marrow dose because the bone marrow is widely distributed throughout the skeleton. The average bone marrow dose in the United States from medical radiation exposure is about 90 mrem/year. Of this, diagnostic x-rays would account for about 72 mrem, dental x-rays contributing 3 mrem and radiopharmaceuticals accounting for another 15 mrem.

The average skin dose from a single chest radiograph is about 25 mrem, with an average bone marrow dose as low as 3 mrem. A barium enema study could deliver a bone marrow dose of 875 mrem/study. All other sources of radiation exposure such as fallout, occupational exposure and releases from the nuclear industry account for less than 2% of the average exposure in the United States.

Maximum Permissible Dose (MPD)

The maximum levels of exposure of radiation workers and the general public have been established by several national and international scientific organizations, such as the International Commission on Radiologic Protection (ICRP) and the National Council on Radiation Protection and Measurement (NCRP). The maximum permissible dose (MPD) is the highest dose of ionizing radiation from both internal and external sources that is not expected to cause appreciable bodily damage to a person at any time during his or her lifetime. Different standards apply for occupational conditions and for the whole population. A radiation worker would be any individual engaged in an occupation involving the use of x-rays, radioactive substances or nuclear reactors. For this group somatic affects rather than genetic hazards are of principle concern. Because of the risks of late effects of ionizing radiation, no matter how remote, the ALARA principle should be applied - radiation exposure should be kept as low as reasonably achievable.

Table 19.2
MPD Occupational Exposure

Site	MPD
Whole body	3000 mrem/quarter year
Skin of whole body	7500 mrem/quarter year
Hands, forearm, feet, ankles	18,700 mrem/quarter year

The long-term accumulated MPD whole body dose in mremsis limited by the formula 5000 x (n-18), where n equals the age of the worker in years. Thus, persons under 18 years or younger are not permitted to be occupationally exposed. Special precautions are taken in the case of pregnant women who are occupationally exposed with the MPD limited to 500 mrem to the fetus for the entire gestation. The scientific councils who advise about MPD's do not forbid pregnant nurses or physicians to care for patients containing therapeutic amounts of radioisotopes, although this is the policy of some hospitals.

MPD General Public

The exposure of a single member of the general public should be limited to 500 mrem/year according to NCRP recommendations. The recommended average dose rate for the general public is 107 mrem/year.

RADIATION SAFETY OFFICER

Any institution involved in the use of radioactive sources customarily assigns an individual known as the radiation safety officer to oversee their safe handling and use. This person is charged with the following responsibilities: (1) awareness of radiation safety regulations and restrictions imposed by both federal and state authorities, (2) insuring that individuals are qualified to use various radioactive materials and that their exposure does not exceed MPD, (3) monitoring of the safety of the working environment, (4) carrying out prepared localization and decontamination procedures should spillage of radioactive material occur, (5) insuring proper disposal of radioactive waste and (6) keeping accurate records which may extend over many years.

MONITORING

Area Monitoring

1. Treatment rooms housing sources such as a cobalt teletherapy unit or a linear accelerator contain permanently installed monitors which would warn a person entering the room if there was a high level of radiation present due to machine malfunction.

2. Portable survey meters are also useful in monitoring rooms where procedures involving radioactive sources have been carried out, namely the operating room or the patient's hospital room in the case of intracavitary or interstitial implants using afterloading techniques.

Personnel Monitoring

This is carried out to determine the radiation dose received by the whole body or one part that might be more heavily exposed. X-ray film badges are most commonly employed because of their convenience and inexpense. These provide a permanent record of exposure and should be worn by any one working with isotopes or with radiation oncology patients in whom permanent or temporary radiation sources have been placed. Ring badges that contain crystals sensitive to ionizing radiation may also be worn by personnel who directly handle radiation sources. There is, however, a delay in film processing which may not be acceptable in cases when exposures are varying rapidly or may be high. In this case, pocket dosimeters or pocket ion chambers are the preferred method. The pocket dosimeters are small ionization chambers with built in electroscopes and optical magnifying systems which can be read immediately by the exposed person. Pocket ion chambers must be read by the use of an auxillary electrometer, usually by a responsible member of the radiation safety office who can interpret the readings and take appropriate action.

Sometimes it is necessary to monitor exposure to radiosensitive organs or tissues of a patient during the administration of therapuetic doses of external beam radiation. This can best be accomplished by using thermoluminescent dosimeters (TLD). These are disks, rods or chips made of crystals (e.g. LiF) sensitive to ionizing radiation. These can be applied to the skin or inserted into a body cavity. After the treatment is delivered with the TLDs in place, the crystals are then analyzed and the absorbed radiation dose in rad is derived from a standard calibration curve. This technique is valuable in verifying the calculated dose to a radiosensitive structure such as the eye.

PRINCIPLES OF RADIATION PROTECTION

Once the source of ionizing radiation has been identified, exposure hazards to humans can be reduced or eliminated by employing any or all of the following safeguards:

1. Distance: The further a person is away from a radiation source, the less will be his exposure (see Inverse Square Law, Chapter 1).
2. Time: The total radiation exposure is equal to the exposure rate times the amount of time one is exposed to a radiation source; therefore, by limiting the time of exposure one can diminish one's total dose.
3. Shielding: The intensity of radiation can be diminished by interposing barriers of appropriate thickness. The concept of half value layer was previously discussed and equals the thickness of an absorber, which reduces beam intensity to one-half its original value.

Diagnostic radiologists use thin lead aprons to protect themselves or personnel during fluoroscopic procedures. These are adequate to markedly diminish exposure to scattered x-rays in the 50-100 KeV range, which are produced during such procedures. The amount of lead needed to reduce exposure by even one-half for some of the isotopes used in brachytherapy such as gold-198 and cesium-137, would be too heavy for the operator to wear.

These three essential principles of radiation safety, distance, time and shielding, must be considered whenever working with radioactive sources. They must be used sensibly to minimize exposure. For example, if the use of cumbersome shielding makes a procedure more time-consuming, it can negate its purpose. An operator may use less cumbersome shielding so the procedure can be performed more rapidly and thus result in less overall radiation exposure.

Afterloading

The concept of afterloading was introduced to further minimize exposure to operators during brachytherapy procedures. Using afterloading devices allows the placement of the applicator, which contains no radioactivity in an unhurried fashion. Localization films can then be taken with "dummy" sources in place. Computer assisted calculations can be performed to determine the optimum placement of active sources and the time for which they must be left in place. When the patient is back in his or her hospital room, the radioactive sources can be transported to the patient's room in a shielded container and then inserted into the device, minimizing exposure to the radiation oncologist, x-ray technician, O.R. and transport personnel.

Radium Substitutes

The traditional material used for brachytherapy has been radium-226. There are certain hazards associated with the use of encapsulated radium salts. In the decay process radium becomes radon-222, a radioactive gas which presents a special contamination problem should the source rupture during handling. Although this is a rare event, several incidences have occurred. The half-life of radium (1620 years) makes decontamination a major problem. In recent decades, several substitutes including cesium-137, gold-198, iodine-125 and iridium-192 have become available as replacements for radium and radon. None of these isotopes has a gaseous radioactive decay product. The half-lives are much shorter being 30 years, 2.7 days, 60 days and 75 days respectively. Finally, the half-value layers for these isotopes are much less than radium, being 6.5 mm of lead for cesium-137, 2.5 mm for gold-198, 0.4 mm for iodine-125 and 3 mm for iridium-192. Thus, less shielding is required.

Contamination

Accidents involving the handling of radioactive material occasionally occur. The seriousness of such an accident will depend upon the type and quantity of the radioisotope involved. The preplanned response to such possible accidents is the duty of the radiation safety officer. The protection of personnel is of primary concern. The proper management of ventilation systems can minimize the degree of contamination, but this is often impractical to implement.

Should a radioactive liquid be spilled, certain steps must be taken to limit the spread of contamination. Personnel should be careful not to touch wet material with bare hands. Paper towels are used to cover the spill in an effort to contain it. If a person or his clothing has been contaminated, the clothing must be immediately removed and the contaminated skin thoroughly scrubbed. Again, contaminated items should not be handled directly but rather manipulated with forceps. All contaminated material is deposited in the containers designated for radioactive waste. Using damp rags, the surface on which the radioactive material was spilled is washed in an inward spiraling fashion. An effort is made to reduce radioactivity to 5 to 10 times the background counts.

Waste Disposal

When radiopharmaceuticals are used for diagnostic or therapeutic purposes, inevitably waste products are generated. The safe disposal of this waste material is imperative. Depending on the type of waste material and the half-life of the contaminating radioisotope, there are several disposal options:

1. For liquid waste, disposal through the municipal sewer system is acceptable provided the waste material is diluted with an appropriate amount of uncontaminated water. Thus, a patient who has received therapeutic doses of iodine-131 can urinate into the toilet in the patient's hospital room, which is then flushed several times.
2. Storage of contaminated solid materials such as syringes and soiled linen is an option if the contaminating isotope has a relatively short half life. For instance, syringes contaminated with I-131 with its physical half-life of 8 days must be stored in a shielded area for approximately 2 1/2 months (10 half-lives).

Care of the Patient Receiving Brachytherapy

Patients who are administered intravenous or oral doses of radioisotopes become radioactive, as do patients receiving permanent interstitial radioactive implants. Patients who are receiving temporary intracavitary or interstitial radioactive implants are radioactive only while this material is in place. For those patients who have received oral or intravenous administration of gamma-emitting radioisotopes in doses greater than 30 mCi, hospitalization is usually required. Formerly, colloidal gold-198 was used for intracavitary instillations and because of its gamma emissions the same precautions would apply. No such precaution would be necessary for intracavitary instillations of P-32, a pure beta emitter. The present Nuclear Regulatory Commission regulations state that <u>the exposure rate measured at 1 meter must be below 1.8 mr/hour before it is permissible to discharge an iodine-131 patient from the hospital</u>. Radiation safety personnel will monitor such patients on a daily basis.

Vomitus and excreta from patients who have received iodine-131 are radioactive. These may be disposed of through the municipal sewer system.

Patients who have received a <u>permanent iodine-125 implant</u> for tumors of the prostate, pancreas or other sites pose <u>little radiation hazard</u> to personnel because of low energy of the x-rays and gamma rays emitted from iodine-125 (about 30 KeV). Occasionally, the patient who has received IV or oral radioisotopes or a permanent radioactive implant requires emergency surgery. If the amount of isotope does not exceed 5 mCi of any radioactive material, no radiation hazard is present for surgery. If the activity is greater than 5 mCi, the radiation therapist and radiation safety officer should be advised of the planned procedure for further advice. Similarly, if such a patient expires, consideration must be given to the radioisotope content in assessing the exposure risk to personnel for autopsying and embalming the body. If the isotope is less than 30 mCi, embalming may be carried out. If more than 30 mCi activity is present, embalming should be performed in the hospital morgue with a radiation safety officer in attendance.

REFERENCES

1. Recommendations of the ICRP (adopted Jan. 1977), ICRP publication No.26, Pergamon, Oxford (1977).
2. Sources and effects of ionizing radiation, 1977 report by the United Nations Scientific Comittee on the effects of atomic radiation (UNSCEAR) to the General Assembly, United Nations, New York (1977).
3. Natural background radiation in the United States, National Council on Radiological Protection (NCRP Report No. 45), Washington, D.C.
4. Radiation Protection Procedures, Safety Series No. 38, IAEA, Vienna (1973).
5. The effects on population of exposure to low levels of ionizing radiation, Report of the Advisory Committee on the Biological Effects of Ionizing Radiations, National Academy of Sciences, National Research Council, Washington, D.C. (November 1972).
6. Cohn B: The cancer risk from low-level radiation. Health Physics 39:659-678, 1980.
7. Upton AC: The biological effects of low-level ionizing radiation. Scientific American 246:41-49, 1982.
8. Meurk ML and Gorson RO: Radiation Safety in Brachytherapy. Report of the Western Center for Radiologigcal Physics, West Coast Cancer Foundation, San Francisco, California (1983).

Chapter 20

New Developments in Therapeutic Radiology

OVERVIEW

Technological developments in radiation therapy over the past 30 years have contributed greatly to improving the radiotherapists ability to cure cancer. Research in the field of radiobiology has provided a better understanding of the effects of radiation on cells and multiple clinical investigations are presently underway based on results of radiobiologic research. This chapter presents a brief outline of several technical, radiobiologic and immunologic developments in radiotherapy.

INTRAOPERATIVE RADIOTHERAPY

The attraction of intraoperative radiotherapy lies in the direct application of the radiation beam onto the surgically exposed tumor. This permits accurate and precise tumor localization while sensitive normal tissue such as small bowel can be displaced outside the path of the beam. Intraoperative radiation, frequently employing an electron beam, may be used to eradicate unresectable tumors or as an adjuvant to destroy microscopic tumor left behind following resection.

Although Howard University and Massachusetts General Hospital have led U.S. efforts in intraoperative radiotherapy, most of the pioneering work done in the last decade has been carried out in Japan. The cancers most frequently treated have been stomach, bladder and pancreas, but many other cancers have also been treated. Palliation can often be achieved in advanced unresectable tumors. At present there are not sufficient details available to draw conclusions regarding the value of intraoperative radiotherapy as an adjuvant to surgery. Many investigators feel that the greatest contribution of intraoperative radiotherapy to cancer management will probably be in an adjuvant capacity, possibly enabling more limited surgery to be performed.

PARTICLE BEAM RADIATION

Clinical investigations of the value of fast neutrons are now ongoing. Proton beam radiotherapy is also being clinically studied, although on a smaller scale than neutrons. Investigation of other atomic and subatomic particles, primarily pi-mesons and heavy ions, is generally limited to physics facilities.

Neutrons: The main advantage of neutron radiation lies in its greater effectiveness against hypoxic cells than photon radiation, since neutrons are less dependent on oxygen for cell killing. Other potential advantages of neutrons include less variation in radiosensitivity with cell cycle phase and less repair of radiation-induced damage. The clinical relevance of these potential advantages depends on the extent to which they are advantageous in producing tumor damage but not normal tissue damage.

A major disadvantage to date of neutron radiotherapy has been in the poor dose distributions obtainable with available equipment. Many units have had depth dose distributions no better than orthovoltage x-ray units. New high energy cyclotrons and deuterium-tritium generators have been developed to deliver clinically useful neutron beams with dose distributions and other treatment characteristics similar to modern Cobalt-60 units. Neutron treatment is being investigated in England, Holland, Germany, Japan and the United States with an estimated 4000 patients treated worldwide in 1980. In the United States, the National Cancer Institute has embarked on a program to study the clinical usefulness of neutron radiation. Four hospital based treatment facilities have been designated: The Fox Chase Center/University of Pennsylvania in Philadelphia, the M.D. Anderson Hospital in Houston, the University of Washington in Seattle and the University of California at Los Angeles. Neutron treatment of advanced tumors of the head and neck, pelvis and brain are some of several tumor sites under investigation.

Protons: The potential advantage of proton irradiation lies in improved dose localization. The high dose zone of the proton beam, known as the Bragg peak, can be directed accurately and precisely onto the tumor. The beam has sharp distal fall-off and limited scatter so that normal tissue dose is minimized. The Massachusetts General Hospital has used proton beam radiotherapy since the mid 1960's. Although a variety of tumors have been treated with proton beam radiotherapy, the majority have been choroidal melanomas and pituitary tumors. Cranial arteriovenous malformations have also been successfully treated.

ALTERED FRACTIONATION SCHEDULES

Standard radiation fractionation (single daily fractions, 5 days weekly) may not represent optimal treatment to obtain maximal tumor cell kill and minimal normal tissue morbidity. Two approaches in investigating nonstandard fractionation include changing the overall treatment time and changing the number (and size) of daily fractions.

Overall treatment times may be either extended or shortened. Extended overall treatment times, which offer the advantage of sparing some acute radiation morbidity and allowing reoxygenation of hypoxic tumor, could result in decreased tumor control due to tumor cell proliferation. Shortened overall treatment times may be appropriate for rapidly growing tumors to avoid their escaping control due to short doubling times. Radiotherapy schedules employing shortened overall treatment times are referred to as accelerated fractionation.

An increase in the number and reduction in size of daily dose fractions is referred to as hyperfractionation. Using smaller fractions may result in a relative sparing of late radiation effects compared to acute effects without diminishing tumor control. Using short interfraction intervals of 3-6 hours rather than 24 hours results in a relative increase in repair of radiation damage by normal tissues over hypoxic tumor tissues. Preliminary studies of hyperfractionation have been promising. A major cooperative group, the Radiation Therapy Oncology Group (RTOG), is presently conducting several studies to determine its effectiveness in the treatment of tumors of the brain (glioblastoma), head and neck, bladder and breast among other tumors.

RADIATION SENSITIZERS

Radiosensitizers are chemical agents which increase the lethality of radiation when given concurrently with radiation. Oxygen is the most important radiosensitizer known. Some but not all clincial trials using hyperbaric oxygen to diminish tumor hypoxia during irradiation have resulted in improved tumor control. Considerable inconvenience and difficulties are involved administering radiation to patients in a hyperbaric oxygen chamber. There have been no recent investigations of hyperbaric oxygen.

A search for a substitute for oxygen as a radiosensitizer has led to the discovery of several potentially useful compounds. In general, compounds which are electron affinic appear to be effective radiation sensitizers. The nitroimidazoles, misonidazole and metronidazole (Flagyl), have been clinically investigated as radiosensitizers. Flagyl has not been found to be a potent radiosensitizer in a clinical setting. Misonidazole administered orally at relatively high doses has resulted in improvement in local tumor control, but toxicity exists at such doses (peripheral neuropathy, nausea and rare encephalopathy). This toxicity has limited the dose of misonidazole that can be administered to less than effective levels for radiosensitazation. Other compounds such as SR-2508 are currently under investigation.

RADIATION PROTECTORS

Sulfhydryl compounds have been shown to be effective radiation protectors. The mechanism by which they exert their protective effect is not clearly understood. Protectors are being developed which offer promise of differentially protecting normal tissues over tumors. A compound, WR-2721 (a thiophosphate derivative of cysteamine), is currently under clinical investigation.

HYPERTHERMIA

There is a firm biologic basis for the use of hyperthermia in oncology. Using cell culture techniques, cell survival curves similar to those achieved for ionizing radiation have been generated following exposure of mammalian cells to various temperatures for varying periods of time. The mechanisms for hyperthermia-induced cyto-toxicity are not well defined but may be related to the following factors:

1. Irreversible damage to cellular respiration.
2. Alterations in nuclear acid and protein synthesis.
3. Increase in cell membrane permeability.
4. Liberation of lysozymes.

Objective tumor responses to hyperthermia alone certainly occur but most of these are only partial and are short-lived. A synergistic interaction between radiation and hyperthermia can be demonstrated whether the heating preceeds or follows irradiation. This effect is believed to be due to hyperthermia-induced inhibition of cellular recovery from sublethal radiation damage. Another rationale for combining the two modalities is that the radioresistant hypoxic component of some tumors is poorly vascularized with an acidic pH - two factors making these cells more susceptible to thermal killing. Also, cells in the radioresistant "S" phase are quite vulnerable to heat.

Clinically, hyperthermia has been applied locally, regionally and systemically. A variety of techniques are presently available to accomplish local heating and include:

1. Interstitial hyperthermia using low frequency current fields applied between implanted electrodes (resistive heating)
2. Interstitial microwave heating using implanted antennae (near field effect)
3. Externally applied microwaves using frequencies ranging from 100 MHz to 2450 MHz
4. Ultrasound
5. Radiofrequency heating at 13.56 MHz and 27.1 MHz
6. Capacitive electrodes
7. Magnetic induction coils or loops

All of these techniques have their theoretical advantages and limitations.

A wealth of clinical experience with hyperthermia in the treatment of superficial malignancies such as metastatic cancer involving cervical nodes, melanomas and locally recurrent breast cancer has been accumulated at several centers in the United States. Using modest doses of radiation (1600-1400 rad), complete responses have been reported in 40-80% of patients treated with combined radiation-hyperthermia. An additional 20-40% will have partial responses (> 50% regression). Normal tissue tolerance is similar to that seen with radiation alone. The Thermal Enhancement Ratio (TER), the ratio of radiation dose required to elicit a certain end-point when given alone to the dose when given with hyperthermia, has been shown to be in the of 1.4.

RADIOISOTOPIC IMMUNOTHERAPY

Antibodies directed against tumor-associated or tumor-specific antigens provide a means of delivering radioisotopes to tumor deposits throughout the body for the diagnosis and treatment of malignant disease. The targeting of tumor deposits with isotopic immunoglobulins in essence represents a "biologic implant". In addition to the cytotoxic effects of the radiation delivered to tumor, secondary immunologic phenomenon may also be elicited resulting in tumor clearance by the host immune system. The use of antibodies to serve as carriers for cellular toxins and chemotherapeutic agents is also being investigated. Two classes of IGG immunoglobulins, polyclonal and monoclonal, are available for clinical use.

The Radiation Therapy Oncology Group has recently completed a phase II study of isotopic immunologlobulin in the integrated multimodal treatment for primary hepatocellular carcinoma under the direction of Dr. Stanley Order at Johns Hopkins Hospital. Toxicity was restricted to the hematopoietic system as dose-related leukopenia and thrombocytopenia occurred 4-6 weeks after eah administration of radioantibody. A partial response rate of 48% was obtained with stabilization of disease in another 28%. The median survival for the non-AFP positive hepatomas was approximately one year with several long-term remissions achieved. The RTOG will shortly compare the use of radiolabeled antibodies against adriamycin and 5-FU chemotherapy in the treatment of hepatocellular carcinoma in a phase III randomized study. There are several other ongoing studies investigating the role of immunoglobulins in the treatment of unresectable non-oat cell lung cancer and advanced Hodgkin's disease which has proved refractory to MOPP and ABVD chemotherapy.

REFERENCES

1. Goldson A.: Past, present and prospects in intra-radiotherapy. Semin Oncol 8:59-64, 1981.
2. Catterall M: The assessment of the results of neutron therapy. I J Rad Onc Bio Phys 8:1573-1580, 1983.
3. Kjellberg R, et al: Bragg-peak proton-beam therapy for arteriovenous malformations of the brain. N Eng J Med 309:269-273, 1983.
4. Peschel R and Fischer J: Optimization of the time-dose relationship. Semin Oncol 8:38-48, 1980.
5. Philips T: Sensitizers and protectors in clinical oncology. Semin Oncol 8:65-82, 1980.
6. Storm FK and Morton DL: Localized hyperthermia in the treatment of cancer. CA 33:44-56, 1983.
7. Order SE: Monoclonal antibodies: potential role in radiation therapy and oncology. I J Rad Onc Bio Phys 8:1193-1201, 1982.
8. Leichner PK et al: Dosimetry of 131-I-labelled antiferritin in hepatoma: specific activities in tumor and liver. Cancer Treatment Reports 67:647-654, 1983.

Index